Latest Combinations for Homeopathy

(Low Potency- High Results)

By

Dr. Balaji Deekshitulu P V

D.II.M.S, B.A.S.M (Alt.Medi), MSc (Psy), PhD, DLitt (USA)

(Homeopathy & Alt. medi physician)

Publication

Amazon, USA

Foreword

It gives me great pleasure to contribute a foreword to yet the book from the versatile pen of Dr. Balaji Deekshitulu, who has practiced diligently for the past 10 years as Alternative Medicine (Homeopathy) Consultant and Psychologist in the Sri Balaji Homeo Clinic, Tirupati. He has treated over a thousands of patients his indeed, is a mature experience which he passes on to his colleagues & students and public through 44 research publications & 3 books, seminars, articles in various magazines and news papers.

The book comprises of several homeopathic combinations for various diseases. In addition, the book consists of case studies which will help the readers understand the usage of different homeopathic medicines. This book is essential for beginners who have just started practice and experienced professionals.

The book will undoubtedly be a boon to all categories of latest combinations in homeopathy in all diseases and will help them to grasp precisely the intricate concepts of this useful of homeopathy remedies, and also help own practical easy methods non side effects way. This book exhibits a rare clarity of thinking and precise approach in explaining the world uniquie combinations in homeopathy for all sitituations, I fervently hope that outstanding success is now within your reach –the keys to achieving it are in your hands!

Combination homeopathic remedies are safe, effective and compatible with all types of medical, surgical, psychological, physical and nutritional therapies; Homeopathy is safe for treating infants, children, elderly patients and individuals. Homeopathy stimulates the body into a healing process - it goes beyond treating the symptoms, and helps the patient heal completely Combination homeopathy is easy to learn and use.

Finally I remembering & i would like to express my heart full thanks for my Grand father, Teacher & Philosher Homeopathic Doctor Late Dr.T.Hanumatharao Garu & great Ayurvedic & Homeopathic Doctors Lt. Dr. Alahari Venkatacharyulu Garu & Lt. Dr. V. Krishnamacharyulu Garu & Devaih garu and lastly my sincear thanks to my PhD Guide, great Psychologist & Legend Dr.B.V.Pattabhi Ram Garu.

Dr. Balaji Deekshitulu P V

Contents

This book is dedicated to
P.Seetharama charyulu& Lakshmi
(My Father& Mother)

Note: only give me Low potencies 30 or 200 selected one are two common medicines on diagnosis basic.

<u>MIND SYMPTOMS</u>

- **Absent mind:** Lac c
- **Abusive:** Kali i
- **Anger:** Ant c, Acon
- **Aversion:** Adren, Kali p, Nat m, Nat ar
- **Cheating:** Puls, Coca
- **Confedence:** Anac (lack of self confedince), Cimic (Confusion of mind), Aur (very exetable), Anthraci & Lac d (Depression), Nat s (Dpressive thoughts of sucide), Ambr (violent temper), Agar (irritability), Acetanilidum (very tried).
- **Desire:** Calad (Erections), Agn, Ambr (violent morning erections), Lac c (no desire to live), Am c (great desire to sugar), Lac felinum (great desire to eat paper), Absin (frequent desire to urinate), Lac d (all types of desires), Electric (dead).
- **Eating:** Abrot (agrgravation after eating, drinking, vomting and stool),
- **Fear:** Acon (Death) & Phos
- **Frightened:** Phos, Lac c, Ambr
- **Hallucinations:** Absin (loss of consciousness, audio –visual), Act sp (hate solitude), Lac c(writing make mistakes).
- **Hurry:** Acon
- **Impulse:** Acon
- **Insanity:** Bac & Apis (joyless)
- **Irritability:** Ambr, Kalip, Aesc
- **Laughing:** Ambr
- **Jealousy:** Hyoscy, Laches, Nat m, Plat m.
- **Love:** Cimic
- **Memory:** Ambr
- **Nervousness:** Ambr, Nat ar, Cimic

- **Nymphomania:** Ambr
- **Offended:** Aur
- **Playfull:** Diph,
- **Prostation:** Acon, Gelsi, Agar.
- **Pulling:** Lac d
- **Quarrelsome:** Acon
- **Recognize:** Ars
- **Sadness:** Agn
- **Shy:** Kali p
- **Speech:** Elec
- **Spit:** Acon
- **Suicidal:** Ciomic
- **Suspicious:** Anthar
- **Sympathetic:** Cimic
- **Talking:** Ambr
- **Weeping:** Ambr & Nat m
- **Wrong:** Kali c & Abies c
- **Worry:** Acon, Ign, Kali p
- **Mental shock:** Apis, Acon, Agar, Ambr
- **Memory:** Anac (week), Agar (slow), Ambr (impaired), Acet ac (mistakes in speking), Agn & Ailanthus gland (loss of memory), Aesc, Bell, Lac d.
- **Mania:** Cann I, Canth, Hyos, Cimic, Bell, Ars, Absin, Veart, Am cx, Anac.
- **Moods:** Anti c, Crotalus, Ig, Nux m, Puls, Saras, Terent,

MENTAL HEALTH

- **Insomnia, Sleeplessness, Sleep Disorders:** Nux vomica, Opium, Coffea cruda, Ambra grisea, Hyoscyamus niger, Sulphur, Belladonna, Chamomilla, Arsenic album, Argenticum nitricum, Gelsemium, Ignatia amara, Magnesium carbonica, Cocculus indica, Aconitum napellus, Arnica Montana, Causticum, Ferrum metallicum, Muriaticum acidum, Tabacum, Senecio jacobaea, Cannabis indica, Kalium phosphoricum.

- **Mood Disorders, Depression, Mania, Bipolar Disorder:** Anacardium, Belladonna, Stramonium, Arsenic album, Hyoscyamus, Carcinosin; Lachesis; Medorrhinum; Staphysagria; Psorinum; Argentum Met; Aurum Met; Platina; Thuja; Sepia; Agaricus; Rhus Tox; Cimicifuga; Causticum and many other medicines.

- **Obsessive Compulsive Disorder OCD:** Arsenic album,Cannabis indica, Lachesis, Medorrhinum, Natrum mur,Pulsatilla, Rhus-tox,Carcinocin etc

- **Psychological Disorders:** Belladonna. [Bell] , Hyoscyamus. [Hyos] , Stramonium. [Stram], Aurum metallicum. [Aur], Sulphur. [Sulph]

- **Anxiety and stress:** Argentum Nitricum, Arsenicum Album, Ignatia Amara, Phosphorus, Gelsemium Sempervirens, Aconitum Napellus, Nux Vomica

- **ADHD:** Stramoni,Cina and Hyos, Lyssi

- **Epilepsy**: Calcarea carbonica, Bufo rana, Cuprum Metallicum, OEnanthe crocata, Kali bromatum, Silicea, Hyoscyamus.

- **Schizophrenia:** Lachesis, Ars-alb, Aurum-met, Hyoscyamus, Lycopodium, Pulsatilla, Stramonium, Sulphur, Aconite, Belladona, Ignatia, Merc-sol, Psorinum, Rhus-tox, Anacardium,Calc-carb, Causticum, Cimicifuga, Helleborus, Kali-brom, Natrum-sulph, Opium, Sepia, Aurum-mur, Cannabis-indica etc.

- **Phobia:** Aconite, Stramonium, Opium, Nux vom, Cuprum met, Mercurius, Cuprum aceticum, Calcaria Carb, Hyoscyamus, Succinum, Ignatia, Gelsemium, Argentum Nitricum, Lyssin.

- **Stress:** Aconite, Calcaria Carb, Lycopodium, Nux vom.

- **Mental weakness**: Arg. n., Nux v., Sil.

- **Hysterical (clavus)** -- Agar., Aquil., Coff., Euonym., Hep., Ign., Kali c., Mag. m., Nat. m., Nux v., Plat., Puls., Thuja.

- **Emotional disturbances**: Acetan., Arg. n., Cham., Cim., Coff., Epiph., Gels., Ign., Mez., Phos. ac., Picr. ac., Plat., Rhus t., Sil.

- **Tension** - Acon., Arn., Asar., *Bapt.*, Canchal., Caust., Iris, Merc., Paris, Ratanh., Selen., Sticta, Viola.

HEAD TROUBLES

Alopecia/Bladness: Nat m, Vinc, Bac, Fl ac, Phos, Weis, Ph ac,Graph, Sep.

Burning: Alumen, Acon, Apis, Alum, Auram, Bell, Glon, Helon, Lach, Rhus.t, Sul, Tarx.

Bursting: Acon, Bell, Bry, Caps, China, Gels, Glon, Lach, Lit.t,Nat.m, Nux.v, Puls, Sep, Veart.a.

Dandruff: Badiga, Lac c, Thuja, Phos, Ars, Kali. Bi, Vinc, Lyco, Graph, Kali.s,

Headache: Bell, Ptel, Gels, Chion, Sep, Sang, Spig, Usnea barbata, Cimic,Nat m.

Hysteria: Agri m, Amm c, Asafoetida, Campho, Cimici, Cinamomum, Conium, Hyosc, Ig, Kali p, Kresot, Moschus, Nat m, Platinum m, Pothos, Tarentula, Thyrodi, Valerian, Viola oda, Zinc val.

Itching: Alum, Ant c, Ars, Bov, Cal c, ,Cleam, Graph, Nit.ac, Nat.m, Oleand, Sep, Sil, Sulf, Vinc

Lice: Bac,Carb ac, Vinc.m, Graph, Nat.m, Staph,, Psori, Lyc.

Migraine: Alfa alfa, Arg.n, Avena, Bell, Cim, Coff, Gels, Iris, Nux.v, Puls, Sang, Sep, Stann, Damiana.

Menstruation: Bell, Bry, Cim, Crocus, Graph, Kali.p, Lac.def, Nat.m, Pul, Sep, Sul.

Neurology top head: Cimi,Gels, Glon, Acon, Bell, China s,Mag p.

Nervous: Anac, Arg.n, Cim, Gels, Ign, Kali.p, Mag.p, Nux.v, Phos.ac, Picr.ac, Sil, Zinc.m.

Spinal: Alfa alfa, Avena, Bell, Bry,Carb.v, Cim, Cocc,Eup.perf, Gels, Nat.m, Nux.v,Petro, Phos ac, Pic.ac,, Sang, Sep, Sil.

Stop Hair fall/ Hair growth: Vinc.m,Ph ac, Thal, Sep, Alumia, Aloe, Ambra, Thuj 1M, Thyr.

Vertigo/Giddiness: Alum,Ambra, Ars, Arg nit, Bapt, Bar c, Bar m, Carbo a,Carbo.v, Con, China, Coccul,Eup.perf, Gels, Granat, Hydrast, Iod, Lyco, Nux.m, Opium, Rhus.t, Sec, Selen, Sul.

EYES

Ball removal: Mezereum

Blindness: Caust, Oxytrop, Stram, Dig, Elec, Acon, Bell, Achyra, Arg n

Burning Eyes: Apis, Acon, Ars, Bell, Canth, Euph, Nat m, Puls, Merc c, Sang, Sul.

Black spots: Sulph.

Cataracts: Sulf, Sulf ac, Sepia, Calc c, Cal f, Cadm s, Cine, Caust, Colchi, Cineria.

Chalazion (Eyelid Cyst): Apis, Con, Graph, Hep,Lyco, Puls, Sep,Sil, Staph,Sul,Thuja.

Conjunctivitis (Pink Eye) Acute /Chronic and Blepharitis: Acon, Apis, Agrn, Ars, Alum, Bell, Euph, Heper s, Kali bi,Puls, ,Merc,Thuja, Euphrasia Drops.

Detachment of retina: Napthaline

Double vision: Arn, Aurum,Bell, Cycl, Gels, Hyos, Nat m, Oleand, Plumb, Stram, Verat v

Eyes color blindness: Agar, Phos

Eye lids swollen/ Itching/ Ulcer: Gels, Ars, Euph, Cham, Merc s.

Eyes dimness: Ambra

Far sightedness: Calc c, Nat m, Petrol. Pilocarpus, Ruta, Sep.

Glaucoma: Osmium met, Phos, Physostgma, Sil, Spigi, Cedr, Gelsi

Hemianopia: Aur met (upper half visible), Lyco(Left half), Mur ac(vertical half)

Itching: Acon,Apis, Arg n, Bell, Euph, Hep s, Kail bi, Meze, Alum g, Fago.

Iritis: Colocynth, Heper sul, Merc sol.Nit ac, Rhus t, Symphytum.

Letters Run: Agar, Bell, Calc c, Cina, Cand ind,China, Con, Hyos, Lyco, Nat m, Sil.

Myopia (short sight): Carb sul, Physostigma, Pilocarpus.

Night blindness: Lyco, Physosti, Ranun bul.

Photophobia: Bell, Calc c, Crotalus h, Graph, Merc sol, Nux v, Rhus t, Sili.

Potosis: Alum, Cast, Gels, Helon, Kali,Nit ac, Cocc, Nux v, Plumb, Ruta, Sep,Stram,Verat a, Zin m.

Sty (Stye): Apis,Calc p, Con, Graph, Hep s, Kali iod, Merc, Puls, Sep, Sil, Staph, Lyco, Sul, Thuja.

Sudden loss of vision: Iodum, Acon

Twitching: Agar, Apis, Ars Caust, Cham, Cocc, Ign, Mag p,Nat m, Nux v, Physost, Plat, Puls, Rheum,Sul.

EAR TROUBLES

- **Burning ears:** Acon, Alum, Ars, Arundo, Bell, Caps, Graph, Kreost, Sang, Sul, Tellu.
- **Buzzing ears:** Am c, Anc, Bar c, Bar m,Cast, Chenop, ,China, Graph, Kali m, Nat s, Puls, Sul.
- **Discharge (Otorrhoea):** Cal c, Carb v, Hep, Graph, Kali m, Merc sol, Nat m, Psori, Puls, Sil, Sulf, Thuja.
- **Deafness of ear:** OLD People: Ambra, Amc, Bary c, Bry m, Cast, Chenop, China, Kali m, Lyco, Mulllein oil, Nat s, Crbo s, Graph, Hydras, Iod, Kali bi, Merc d, Nit ac, Puls,Sil.
- **Dullness of hearing:** Ambra, Anac, Aurum, Bell, Cast, China, Gelsi, Ign, Lach, Phos ac, Phos, Plat, Tab, Val.
- **Earache (Otitis/ Otalgia/ Inflammation):** Kali m, Puls, Cham, Merc, Graph, Tell (Eczema), Acon, Ferr p, Kali s, **Bell**, Caps,Hep s.
- **Eczema wet of ear:**Ars, Clem, Cort t, Graph, Mez,Lyc, Merc, Sil,Sul.
- **Glands about ear swell (Mumps):** Abrot, Carb v,Pilo, Rhus t, Bell, Merc, Puls, Aur, Parotodi.
- **Itching of ear:** Bell, Hep, Merc, Sil, Sul.
- **Impaired:** Ambra, Arn, Bryt c, Chenapodium.

NOSE

Adenoids: Calc.c, Merc, Bac, Calc.p, Agrap, Cist, Bar.c, Merc iod, Cal.f, Calc.iod, Tuber, Bacci, Lyco, Sil.

Abscess: Aur m ,Hep s.

Bleeding: Bell, Ferum p, Mill f, Hamamelis Q(Cotton plug), Phos, Bry, Ambra, Amm c, Lyco.

Block: Lyco

Burning: Aurum, Calc.c, Echin, Hep,Hydrast, Kail.bi, Merc s, Sep, Puls,Sul,, Sil.

Itching: Alum, Anac, Bell, Calc.c, Hep, Kali.bi, Mez, Merc s, Nt.m, Nit.ac, Puls,Sul,, Sil.

Odor (smell): Alli cepa, Anthra, Aur m (everthing smell bad), Colchicum (smell of cooking foods), Helleborus (bad mouth), Kali p(breath), mag mur (bad taste), Phos (garlic), Psori(discharge of body). Sul(body),

Pain: Rheum

Polyp: Farmica rusa, Thuja, Tucrum.m.v, Lemnaminor.Calc c,

Running Nose: Hep

FACE

Acne: Anthraci, Berb.a, Ant.c, Calc.s, Sul, Graph, Sang, Thuja

Anemic look: Ars, Calc.c, Calc.p, Ferr.m, China.s, Crataegus Q, Carb.v, Nat.m, Puls, Nux.v, Phos.ac

Boils: Arn, Bell, Sul, Hep, Sil, Echn.

Old man looks: Ambra, Arg.c, Con, Lyco, Carbo v, Helo, Nux.m, Nux.v, Sel, Utrica, Urens Q.

Paralysis: Amm p, Cadmium sul, Caust, Senega.

Pimples: Berb a, Ambr, Adren, Arn, Aur, Bell, Acon, Elec, Lac.d, Abroma Aug.

Skin face cracked: Agra, Alum, Am c, Am m, Ant.t, Ars, Arum.t, Bov, Calc. c, Carbo an, Cham, China, Graph, Lach, Mag m, Nat c, Nat m, Sul.

Swelling in face: Colchicum, Ars a, Vipera

MOUTH

Apthae / Mouth affection : Acid.nit, Merc.s, Hydrs, Borax, Kal.m, Merc.c, Sul.ac, Bapt, Apis, Agar, Carb. v, Anthra.

Bad taste: Puls

Corners of mouth cracked: Aeth, Ant c, Ars, Aurm t, Canth, **Graph**, Hep, **Nat m**, Nit ac, Petrol, Rhus t, Sec, **Merc sol, Puls**.

Jaw: Acid fl, Acon, Helleborus, Hekla lava, Lac can, Phos, Rhus t, Lac can.

Mouth offensive after sleeping: Rheum

Mouth open sleep: Opium

Ulcer: Kali chlo, Bapt (Child).Merc sol (Adults)

<u>TONGUE and TASTE</u>

Inflammation /Swelling: Acon, Apis, Ars, Aurum.t, Bell, Canth Lach, Merc.c, Ox ac, Mur ac, Crot t, Sul ac, Vespa.

Slow lerning/talking and walking: Agar, Bar c, Calc, Calc p, Bell, Bov, Caust, Cann I, Mag c, Mag p, Nat c, Nat m, Nux.v, Sanic, Sil, Stram, Merc.s.

TEETH and GUMS

Bleeding of Gums: Agave, Alum,Ambra, Arg.n Arn, Ars, Borax, Carbo v,,Iod, Kreos, Lach, Merc s, Nit.ac, Plant, Thuj.

Burning: Acon, Arg.n, Bapt, Bell, Calc f, Carb v, Can, Hekla, Hep, Kreso, Merc, Nit.ac, Plant, Sil, Sul, Thuja.

Dentition: Cham, Calc p,Rheum, Kreos, Aeth, Calc.c.

Extraction: Hyper, Artn, Staph, Phos, Trill pend.

Grinding: Bell, Clc, Cina, Physost, Plant, Pod, Santon.

Gum Boil: Alum, Ambra, Arg n, Arn, Ars, Carbo v, Boar, Iod, Kreos, Merc, Nit ac, Plant.

Inflamed Gums: Alum, Arn, Arg n, Bapt, Bell, Bor, Carb v, Hep, Kreos, Merc s, Nit ac, Plant, Sil,Thuja.

Neuralgic toothache: Acon, Ars, Bell, Bry, Carb v, Cham, Coff, Kreos, Mag c, Mag p,Merc,Plat, Puls, Staph,Sil.

Swelling: Pencilin,Merc s.

Toothache: Coff, Staph, Hyos, Clematis, Mag c (Prgnat time toothache), Ars, Plantago, Kreost, Arn, Lac.d (Loss Teeth).

Ulceration: Bapt, Carb v, Caust, Cistus, Hekla, Kroes, Merc c, Merc s, Nit ac, Plant, Sep, Sil, Staph, Thuja.

ENDROCRINE DISORDERS

Acromegaly: Pitutary, Spongia, Thyrodi

Decrease in production of spermatozoa (Sub fertility): Cantha, Nux v.

Decrease in production of estrogen (Masculinization symptoms in women): Cantha, Nux v.

Gynecomastia (Enlargement of mammary glands in male): Merc iod flavus (proto ioduts)

Goitre: Calc iod, Calc c, Iodium, Nat m, Spongia, Thyrodi.

Diabetis: Ars brom, Calc fl, Coca, Phos, Uranium nit, Cephlendra, Syzigum, Insulin, Fungreek, Rudranathri, Ozone, Cantharidinum.

Hormones: Adrenli, Agnus, orchitnum, Tribulus, Insulin, Thyrodi,

Hormonal imbalance womens: Puls, Sep, Laches, Ign, Conium, Nat m,Calc carb,

Hypoglycemia (Low blood sugar): Allumina sil.

Obesity: Calc c, Calc fl, Nat m, Phytolacca, Thyrodinum, fuccus v, Carb apple, amm m, amm p,

Hypothyroid: Bryt iod, Bell, Calc c, Calc fl, Calc iod, Cistus, Ferr p, Iod, Kali c, Kali iod, Petro, Sep, Thyrodi, Tuberc.

Hyperthyroidism: Alnus 3c, Bromi, Echni, Ephedra, Fucus ves, Iod, Lyco, Nat m, Petro.

THROAT

Burning throat: Agr n, Ars, Calc c, Carb v, Hydras, Lyco, Nat c, Nux.v, Puls, Robinia, Sep, Sul, Sul ac.

Choking / Croup: Acon, Broam, Calc fl, Hep, Iod, Ipec, Kali bi, Kali m, Sang, Spang.

Crust/ Mucus adherent in pharynx: Alum, Arg m, Arg n, Aurm t, Calc c, Canth, Carb v, Caust, Coccu, Con, Hep, Hydrast, Kali bi, Kali m, Lach,, Nat m, Nux v, Phyto, Psoi, Sele, Rumex, Sep, Stann,Wyeth.

Swelling and pain: Bapt, Bell, Bry, Canth, Caps, Cic, Hep, Hysosc, Ign, Lach,Merc c, Merc s, Nat p, Nit ac, Phyto.

Deptheria: Acon, Aesc, Apis, Ars, Arum, Bell, Bapt, Canth, Diph, Echin, Hep, Kali m, Lach, Phyto,Nit ac, Vinca,**Amm-c**.

Dryness: Acon, Aesc, Alum, Apis, Ars, Arum, Bell, Bry, Canth, Caps, Cocca, Ferr p, Gels, Guaiac, Hep, Lyco,Mez, Lach, Phyto,Nux m, Phos, Puls, Sabad, Nit ac, Vinca, Sang, Sep,, Spong, Sul, wyeth.

Facues inflammation/Glands of throat Swollen/ Glands of neck swollen: : Bell, Bar c, Bar m, Calc c, Calc f, Calc iod, Calc p, Hep, Brom, Carb v, Cistus, Con, Iod, Kali bi, kali m, Lyco, Merc s, Nat m, Rhus t, Sil, Sul, Thuja.

Goitre: Am m, Apis, Bar iod, Bell, Brom, Calc c, Calc f, Calc iod, Crot c, Fucus, Flouric ac, Hydrast, Iod, Iris, Kali iod, Lapis alb, Nat m, Phyto, Puls, Sil, Spong, Sul, Thyroid.

Glands swollen: Merc c,Hydras.

Infection: Euphr,

Lump feeling (stone in throat)/ Hawking: Alum, Arg m, Arg n, Aurm t, Calc c, Canth, Carb v, Caust, Coccu, Con, Hep, Hydrast, Kali bi, Kali m, Lach,, Nat m, Nux v, Phyto, Psoi, Sele, Rumex, Sep, Stann,Wyeth.

Mumps: Abrotanum, Carb v, Bell, Merc sol, Parotiidinum, Phytollaca, Pilocarpus, Puls, Trifolium.

Myelitis(inflammation of spinal cord): Acon, Arn, Ars alb, Bell, Cupr ars, Hypericum,Plumbgo,Secale cor, Strychinum p.

Ploiomyelitis (Spinal card): Anac, Lathyrus, Angustura, Diph, Bell, Nux v, Rhus t, Gelsi, Plb, Calc

Tonsils: Acon, Am mur, Calc p, Bell, Bar c, Hep, Lach, Lyco, Merc s, Phyto, Psori, Sang n, Sil, Sul, Thuja, and Bacilin. Hepr, Lac c.

Uvulitis: Alumen, Apis, Bell, Caps, Coccus, Hep, Hysosc, Kali bi, Merc c, Merc s, Phyto,, Nux v, Puls, Trifol.

Voice hoarseness: Alum, Arg m, Caust, Hep, Lach, Sul.

LIVER DISEASES

Acidity /Gastric: Calc c,Crbo v,Arg n, Hydr, Nux v, Puls,

Cirrhosis (Liver)/Fatty Liver: Chel, Lyc, Nux v, Phos, Calc c.

Constipation: Blodo, Chinathus, Mag m, Nasturitum

Dropsy: Arg nit, Cardus, Lyco, Nasturtim.

Emaciation (enlargement of liver and spleen): Aceticum ac

Fever: Ferr ars

Food allergy: Aethusa, Ars alb, Bry, Colchi, Fragaria ves, Sul, Thuja.

Food Poisoning: Ars alb, Carb v, Acet ac, Acon, Euph, Agar, Am, Coffe, Hep, Ranb, Eupf,

Headache: Myrica c

Homeopathic Remedies for Liver Enlargement, Hypertrophy, Jaundice, Hepatitis, Gall Stones: Bry, Merc, Podo, Chel, Dig,Nux v, Lyco, Cardu m, Phos, Tarx, Sulf,Cal c.

Hypertrophy: Increase in the number or size of cells in a tissues in body in any way: Lac d, Ambar, Acet ac (stomac walls),Acon (cardic - left fingers),Aur m, Arn, Rhus t, Cact,

Immunisystem: Adonius, Atheusa(glands inflammation), Allium sat (boost immunesystem), Amm c(glands swollen),Ars a(hepetic fever), Bufo(septic orgin), Cannabis sat & Eucalyptus and Hecklava (non cancerous growth), Feer pic (Hordgkin), Hippozaeninum (spleen swelling)Merc sol, Iod, Scrophularia nodasa, Tuber, Vibru op.

Inflammation: Chelidoni, Nat m, Phos, Vipera.

Indigestion: Alum,Cal c, ,Cic, Ign, Nit a,Psori, Sepia.

Liver abscess: Heper sul, Ptelea tri.

Liver spots: Curare, Lyco, Mezer, Nat sulp, Plumbum m.

Spleen: Agar, Iod, Ars, Cean, Chin, Kali p, Calc p, Phos, Caps, Chino.

Swelling: Acet ac, Ptelea tri,

Ulcer: Aescul h,Acetic a, Arg n,Ars a, Grph,Kali bi,Lach, Merc s, Merc c, Nat p, Sul, Med

Vomiting: Ars, Aeth, Carb v.China,Bry, Ipec, Nux v, Puls, Petrol, Verta a,Graph

Weight in Stomach: Abies n,Arg n, Ars, Bism, Bry, Calc c, Cham, China, Graph, Kail bi, Lyco, Nux v, Nux m, Puls, Robina, Sep, Sil.

<u>ABDOMEN, ANUS and STOOL</u>

Abdomen Colic / Burning: Acon, Aloe, Arg n, Ars, Bell, Bry, Carb v, Colo, Lyco, Nux v, Mag p, Canth.

Abdomen Large, Flabby: Am brom, Fucus,Calc, Ars, Calc c, Phyto, Beries, Kali bi,Thyriod

Abdomen Swollen and Hard: Abrot,Aloe, Anac, Arg n, Asaf, Bar c, Bell, Calc c, Carbo v, China, Cham, Cina, Graph, Lyco, Mag c, Mag p, Nat s, Nux v, Opium, Sil, Thuja.

Anus / Fissure / Bowels, Pain / Itching: Aloe,Calc f, Carb v, Graph, Ham, Hydras, Led, Nat m, Nit ac, Petro, Sil, Thuja. CalendQ +EcachQ+HamQ+HydrasQ +Olive oil Apply External.

Anus Prolapsus: Aesc, Aloe, Arn, Bell, Ign, Pod, Sep, Sil, Sul.

Bleeding Fissures: Aesc, Aloe, Alumen, Alum, Arm m, Anac, Arn, Calc f, Collins, Condura, Graph, Ham, Ign, Iod, Kali c, Lyco, Nat m, Nux v, Paeona, Petrol, Phyto, Plat, Plumb, Ratanh, Sedum, Sep, Sil, Sul.Thuja.

Cholera: Ars, Bell, Ipec, Podo, Campho.

Colitis: Thuja,Alumina, Coloc, Abrot, Acet ac, Lyc 10M, But ac, Canth.

Constipation: Alum, Anti c, Hydras, AlfalfaQ+ Aletris Q + Hydras Q+ Gent Q (1:1:1:1:1)=10-20 Drops, Nux v, Phyto, Selen, Sul.

Constipation / Infants children: Aesc, Alum,Ant c, Bry, Calc c, Collin, Hydras,Lyco, Mag m, Nux v, Opium, Pod, Psori, Sanic, Sep, Sil, Verat a.

Diarrhea: Acon,Aeth, Alston, Ant c, Apis, Arg n, Asaf, Bapt, Bell, Bism, Bry, Calcc, Calc p, Camph, Carbo v, Cham, Chaparral,

Chel, China ars,China, Colo,Cupr ars, Cupr m, Cycl, Dulc, Gamb, Gels, Hep, Ipecac, Iris, Liatris, Mag c, Merc, Nat c, Nat s, Nux v, Phos ac, Pod, Puls, Sec, Sep, Sul, Verat a.

Dysentery: Acon,Arn, Aloes, Ars,Arg n, Bapt, Bell, Bry, Canth, Capas, Carbo v, Cham,Colo, Colchi, China, Cupr ars, Ham, Ipecac, Kali bi, Mag c, Merc s, Merc c, Nat ac, Nux v, Pod, Puls, Rhus t, Sul,Torm.

Dysentery old people: Aloes,Anti c, Anti t, Ars, Bapt, Caps, Carbo v, Chaprral, China, Colch, Ham, Lyco, Nit ac, Nux v, Opium, Phos ac, Pod, Sec, Verat a.

Entreralgia: Acon, Arg n, Ars, Bell, Bism, Bry, Carb v, Cham, China ars, Cocca, Colo, Cort h, Cupr ars, Cupr m, Diosc,Lyco, Mag p, Nux v, Pulmb m, Pod, Puls, Verat a, Sul.

Fistula: Bra m, Berb v, Cac c, Calc p, Calc s, Carbo v, Flour ac, Graph, Hydras, Ham, Nit ac, Nux v, Paeonia, Ratanh, sul, Thuja.

Gall Stones: Dioscorea, Colo , Chel , Berb v, Bell, Card m, Chin, Chol, Lyc, Morg, Net s, Verat, Calc c, Phos.

Hemorrhoids: Aesc, Calc f, Collins, Ham, Ign, Mucuna Q, Nux v, Puls, Sul,Wyeth.

Itching Anus: Aesc, Ambra, Alumen, Anac, Anti c, Bar c, Calc c, Caust, Cina, Collins, Graph, Ign, Indigo, Lyco, Med, Nit ac, Paeonia, Ratanh, Sabad, Sul, Teucr.

Hepatitis / Liver Enlarge : Acon., act-sp., anag., anan., apis., ars., ars-i., aur., bapt., bell., bry., calc., camph., cham., carc., card-m., cean., chel., chin., cocc., corn., cupr., dol., hep., hippoz., hydr., ign., iod., kali-c., kali-i., kali-p., lach., lyc., mag-m., mang., merc., merc-d., nat-a., nat-c., nat-m., nat-s., nit-ac., nux-v., phos., phyt., podo., psor., ptel., puls., pyrog., sec., sil., staph., stel., sulph., tab., zing.

Hernia: Lyc, Nux v, Cocc, Carb v, Ars, Tabacum, Plb, Arn, Aur.

Ineffectual urging of stool: Ambra, Alum, Anac, Anti c, Bar c, Card m, Chel, Con, Caust, Graph, Ign, Lyco, Mag m, Nux v, Opium, Plat, Plumb,Sep,Sul.

Jaundice: Chel, Podo

Marasmus: Thyr, Calc p,Aeth, Iod, Nat m, Bar c, Abrot, Ars.

Pain abdomen: Car v, Colo, Ambr, Lyco, Thuj, Am m,Stann, Nit ac.

Rectum-anus: Aesc, Aloe, Apis, Ars, Ars, Carbo v, Caust, Cham, China, Gels, Graph, Ign, Mur ac, Nat m, Nit ac, Nux v, Pod, Puls, Sep, Sil, Sul.

Spleen pain: Agar, Agn, Am m, Ars, Bellis, Calc ars, Card m, Ceananth, China s, Diosc, Helon, Iod, Kali iod, Nat m, Querc.

Stool types: Aesc, Alum, Bry, Graph, Lyco, Nat m,Nux v, Opium, Plat,Plumb, Sep, Sul, Verat a, Selen.

Tympanitis After Typhoid: Agar,Carb v, Asaf, Terbenth, Puls,Lyco, China

Worms: Cina, Allium sativum, Viola tri, Aegle folia, Alumina, Abro, Adon, Aloe, Sil, Tecur.

URINARY TROUBLES

Albuminuria (Inflammation of kidney): Aur c, Canth, Helon, Apis, Kalmia, Ph ac, Colchi, Merc c, Ox ac,

Bladder Pain: Berb, Bell, Terbi, Kali c, Catha, Hydrange arb, **Straph.** Ambar,Chim, Bufo, Dig, Con, Acon,

Bloody urine: Apis, Arn, Catharis, Fucus rel, Hamamel, Millifoli, Terbenth, Vipera.

Burning/ cutting/ tearing: Acon, Arn. Apis, Arg m, Ars, Berb, Bor, Canth, Caps, Lyco, Sul

Irritation (Frequent urination): Nux v, Merc, Bell,Cham, Ign,

Bedwetting (Weakness of bladder): Hepar

Colitis (inflammation of the large intesiness): Allu sat, Aloes, Arg nit, Cadmium sul, Canth, China of, Colchi, Colocynth, Ficus ind, Kalim bich, Lachs, Mag c, Merc c, Selenium, Sepia, Staph, Sul, Terbenth, Thuja,.

Cystitis: Ars, Benz ac, Ber v, Canth, Carb v, Caust, Chimph, Copiva, Cannb sativa, Calc, Eup, Epig, Purp, Fabiana, Hydras, Lyco, Merc c, Nit ac, Pareira, Puls, Sad, Sep, Terbe, Thuja, Uva

Enuresis: Puls, Apis, Hyos, Ac Benz, Canth, Sil, Lac c, Bell, Acon, Alet, Ant c, Caust, Sep, Gels, Cina, Lac d(Drop urine), Rhus aro.

Failure of kidney: Cupr ars (Headech,vertigo,coma), Morph (slow difficult urination),Veart a, Hallebours, Pilocarpinum.

Fissures: Ana c, Anti c, Lyco, Calc fl, Graph, Hepar sul, Malandri, Mang ac, Nat m, Nit ac, Petro, Platin m, Ranunculs bulb, Ratanhia, Sarasap, Sili.

Urethra bleeding: Phos, Hamam, Ambar(yellowish / itching), Staphy(stone)

Urethra swelling: Thuja, Cann sat

Dropsy: Apis, Merc Sol (Feet), Lyco(Liver), China(Weekiness), Kali carb(Chest), Appocynum & Hellebours (Diarrhoea), Ars & Digi (Heart), Acetic acid (Abdomen), Arg phos (Duritic),

Dysuria(Painful Urination):

Polyuria (execs of urine): Phytolacca, Acid phos, Uranium nit, Nux v.Cantha, Cop, Apis(drops), ,Caust(old people), Arg nit (Diabetic with or without)

Pyelitis (inflammation of pelvis of a kidney): Uva ursi

Gravel colic or Renal colic: Arg nit, Aspar, Bell, Benz ac, Ber v, Calc c, Canth, China s, Coccus, Colo, Disco, Epig, Eup purp, Hydrang, Hedeoma, Lith c, Lyco, Nit ac, Nux v, Occimum, Pereira brava, Thalspi, Utrica.

Haematuria (blood urine): Canth, Ham, Terb, Nit ac, Mille f, Apis (burning and bloody), Arn, Lyco, Thlaspi,

Ischuria (Delay urine): Acon, Apis, Arn, Ars, Bell, Canth, Caust, EUP PER, Hyos, Nux v, Poium, Plumb m, Stigm, Tereb,

Nephritis: Apis, Ars, Canth, Kali bro, Acon, Calc, Helon, Cadmium s, Ter

Utrica itching: Nat m.,Rhus t,

Pus and Mucus in urine (Urine colours): Ars, Aspar,Borax, Benz ac, Berb v, Can s, Chimhiph, Dul, Epig, Hep, Kali bi, Lith c, Lyco, Merc c, Sars, Terb, Thalspi, Uva.

Kidny function stopped: Serum angullae, Zingiber

MALE SEXUAL DISORDERS

Balanitis (Inflammation of glans and Penis: Acon, Apis, Arg n, Calad, Can s, Canth, Cop, Cort t, Gels, Jacar, Lyco, Merc sol, Nit ac, Rhus t, Sul, Sil, Thuja.

Coition, Weakness after intercourse: Agar,Agnas, Anac, Arg n, Ars, Avena, Calc c, Can ind, China, Con, Dig, Kali c, Kali p, Kali s, Lyco, Nat p, Nux v, Phos ac, Pic ac, Sabal, Salix n, Sel, Yohimb.

Erethism (Errection of penis) /Spermantorrhoea: Cald, Can in, Dul, Hysosc, Kali bro, Mosch, Nux v, Plat, Lyco, Sele.

Eruption (Penis Itching, sweating of scrotum: Acon, Apis, Calad, Cinnaab, Canth, Con, Cort t, Graph,HammQ+CaladQ for external, Lyco, Merc sol, Nit ac, Rhus t,Fagop, Sel, Sul, Thuja.

Hydrocele (Swelling in the testes and scrotum)/ Orchitis: : Abrot, Aurum m, Rhododendorn (Left sided), Puls (Without swelling Burning and Aching), Graph, Iodum, Arn, Oleum ni (Nuralgia).Mullion oil (Enlarge testicles), Tuber, Apis, Arg nit.

Itching: Bry cab

Impotency: Phos, Thuja, Sel, Agans, China, Lyco, Graph, Caledi (no ogrgans), Tribuls, Yhimbi,Staph, Silex nig, Sabal serc, Nauphar lut,Gensing, Ginkgo.

Masturbation: Staphy, Nux v.

Old men's look: Ambra, Arg c, Con, Lyco, Cab v, Helon,, Nux m, Nux v, Sel, Utrica urenQ.

Penis small: Ignatia, Lyco, Nuphar, Agnus c.

Penis itching: Caust

Penis swelling: Jacarnda, Viola tri

Penis pain/crushing/ burning: Hyper, Kreosot,Nit ac.

Prostatic fluid discharge: Aesc, Agn, Alum, Anac, Arg n, Caladi, Chimaph, Con, Damiana, Lyco, Nux v, Ac pho, Puls, Sabad, Sel, Sul, Thuj.

Prostitutes: Merc c, Bell, Cal s, Staph, Ars, Bapt, Am c, Gels.

Sterility: Phos,Selen, Thuja,Tribulus t, Turnera Q

Testicles: Acid p, Iod, Thyrodi (small & impotency

Testicles swelling /Pain/ hydrocel: Acon, Aur m, Anti c, Arg m, Bryt c, Bell, Bry, Calc c, Clematis (chronic), Conium, Hamame, Lycopus, Merc bin iod, Merc c, Mezerreum, Nuphar luta, Nux v, Olium, Puls, Rhoden, Sabal serc, Sili, Nat mn, Spongi, Zinc m.

FEMALE SEXUAL DISORDERS

Abortion /Miscarriage: Sep & Puls (Habitual), Sabi & Helon (Every 2 and 3 month), Goss (Abortion producing), Arn (Accident), Cham (Emotional disturbance), Syphillinum (2 Aweek in syphilis), Sil (Rickety), Baccil (Tb once a month)

Amenorrhoea (Fat Girls): Acon (Yong), Platina, Caculus (leucorrhoea), Puls, Ferrum m.

Amenorrhoea (absence of menses in dropsy): Apocy.

Burning of uterus and vagina & Dryness of vagina : Ars, Acon, Ambra, Apis, Bell, Calc c, Cath, Carb v, Cim, Con, Graph, Lyco, Merc c, Merc s, Sep, Sul.

Chlorosis anaemia: Nat m, Alumina

Chlorosis green sickness: Mang, Anmti c, Amm c, Ars, Cocculus, Cal c, Lyco, Carb v, China, Ferr m, Phos, Sep, Sul, Puls, Nux v, Nat m, Ign.

Menses during day only: Caust, Cyclamen

Infertility: Aur m, Borax, Coni, Iod,Nat m, Phos, Sep, Sil.

First Meses Delay in young girls: Kallium carb

Leucorrhoea acrid: Nat m, Flour ac, Agar

Pain before Menstruation: Mag p, Chamm, Acid nit(Metrorrhagia)

Burning sensation in Menstruation: Lach, Puls, China,

Menses Short: Euphr

Menses too late too short: Sul

Menses irregularity: Vibru op, Puls, Ashoka,

Menstruation absence: Phos

Menstruation pains in legs: Calc p

Menstruation bleeding from nose and lungs: Phos

Menopause: Lach, Sep, Gelsi (earache), Caulophillum (Arthritis and rheumatism

Metritis: inflammation of utters: Aurum mur nat

Nymphomania (excessive sexual desire in women): Murex, Stram, Gratiola, Lilium,Platina

Ovary – Pain in right: Podo,Naja, Merc sol, Colocy.

Ovary – Pain in left: Nat M,Puls, Sepi, Calc c, Thuja

Ovary fibrous: Calc c, Platina, Staph, Thuj.

Prolepses uteri: Podo, Nux v, Sep, Aloe, Agn,

Sterility Female: Aur m, Alteris f, Sep, borax, Cal c, Iod, Platina, Aur m nat, Con, Nat carb, Phos

Sterility male: Sel, Bufo, Phos, Eup per,

Tumour Ovaries: Apis, **right:** Apis, fl-ac., iod., Lyc., podo, **left** : Lach., podo.

Uleration of OS, cervix, and vagina: Arg m, Arg n, Ars, Aur m n, Carb ac, Flour ac, Graph, Hydras, Hydrocot, Mur ac, Nit ac, Sep, Thuj, Ustil, Vespa.

Vagina: Ambra, Ign.

Yong girls having no menses for months: Sabina, Sabadilla (too late), Sulph, Tubercu(above all faild),Graph,

WOMEN DISEASES

Aversion of coitoion: DanianaQ, Berb vulg, Ign, Onasmodi, Graph.

Bed wetting (enuresis): Aloes, Arg nit, Bell, Benzic ac, Calc c, Causti, Cina, Ferr p, Equiest, Kali m, Mag p, Kali p, Kreost, Lac c, Lyco, Medorr, Plantago, Psorinum, Pulsat, Sabal serc, Secale c, Senega, Sepia, Sul,

Blood clots: Crocus sat, Cyclamen, Thalapsi

Birth control: Puls (before 4 days menses one dose), Nat m 3x (3 days before 3times in menses), Nat m 200 (after menses 3 times 3days),Tests 3x (after menses 2 times 7 days 3 tabs),Cyclmen Q or Jentho jailum Q (after menses stopped 5drops 10days)

Breast Tumors: Phytolacca, Conium,Calc fl, Carbo ani, Asterian rub, Sili, Sarasaparilla, Nit ac.

Cysts: Apis, bov., bufo., canth.,carb-an., coloc., iod., kali-br., lach., merc., murx., plat., prun-s., rhod., rhus-t., thuj.

Dysmenorrhoea: Kreosotum, Sep, Xantho, Mag c, Cocculus, Vibur op, Act r & Mag p (Pain).

Excessive Bleeding: Ficus rel Q+ Hamma Q

Fallopian tubes: Euponium, Laches, Seleni m, Triticum rep (blockage).

Fibroids: Apis., calc., coloc., fl-ac., hep., iod., lach., merc., plat., podo., staph., thuj.

Green Leucorrhoea: Nit ac,

Gonorrhoea: Aco, Puls, Copiva, Kreos, Merc c, Sil, Ars sul flv, Thuj, Cantha.

Inflamation of the Utres: Apis, Ars a, Bry a, Cimicifuga, Gelsi, Hydrocoty, Murex, Sepia, Viscum a.

Iregular Menses: Nat mur,Nux v, Puls, Ferr m, Graph, Tuber.

Leucorrhoea: Am c (burning and pain), Borax, Agn, Kreso, Phos, Ac phos, Sep (yellow & green),

Menorrhoea (Excessive bleeding or prolonged menses): Aletris far (Early menses with pain ,constipation, indigestion, fatigue), Aloes (too early or too long), Helonias, Ipec, Kreoso, Plati m, **Chronic Menorrhoea:** Ars alb, Caulophyllum, Ambra + Bovista+ Sabina

Menses early: Milli

Menses, before Swollen Ovaries: Brom.

Menses, during Swollen Ovaries: Apis, brom., nat-h.

Metrorrhagia (Bleeding between periods): Bovista, Calc sili, Caust, Erigeron, Fer p, Gaph, Medorr, Nit ac, Phos, Visc alb, Trill pend,

Menopouse: Lach, Puls, Sep, Cimicifuga, Lac can, Gelsi, Sul,

Nymphomania (excessive sex interest): Mosch, Murex, Puls, Plat, Asterian rub, Originum, Phos.

Periods prolonged: Chamo, Bell & Erigeron and Sabina (bright red), China (Black), Ustilgo may (dark blood).

Pelvis: Calc p, Cimicifuga, Mag sul, Medorrh, Rhus t, Sepia.

Sterility: Nat c, Upioanum, Sep, Au mur nat, Aletris f, Borax, Pititu, Abroma aug, Ferr m 10M, Nat p 10M, Kali brom, Nat m.

Swollen Ovaries: Alum., apis, ars., atro., bell., brom., bufo., carb-ac., coll., coloc., con.,cub.,goss,graph.,   ham.iod., kali-br., kali-i.,Lach., Lil-t., med., nat-h.,nux-m.,pall.,   staph.,   syph.,   thuja., usti.......

Swollen right Ovaries : Apis., lyc., pall.

Swollen left Ovaries : Brom., carb-ac., graph., kali-br., Lach., lil-t., nat-h.

Tumors: Calc., coc-c., Lyc., nit-ac. **Encysted:** Bar-c., calc., carb-s., graph., kali-c.,   lyc.,   nit-ac.,   rhod., sabin., sep., sil., sulph. **Erectile:**   Ars., carb-an., carb-v., kreos., lach., lyc., nit   ac., phos., plat., sep., sil., sulph., thuj. **Bleeding** : Arn., coc-c., kreos., lach., phos., puls., thuj. **Bleeding blue** : Carb-v. **Burning** : Calc., carb-an., thuj. **Itching** : Nit-ac. **Pricking** : Carb-v. **Sticking** : Nit-ac. **Hard :** Carb-v.

Under growth of breasts: Iod, Sebal serc, Chimphila, Fragrarian vesc, Onasmodi 10 M, Pitutary, Nux m.

Young Girls non development of breasts: Lyco, Pitutary, Sabal serc

Utress Tumors: Aur mur nat, Fractinas am, Trili, Kali iod, Lapis alb, Calc iod, Thuj, Graph, Mill.

Utres Prolapse: Bell, Nux v, Sep, alc c, Lilium t, Calc fl.

Vagina: Kreso (Burning,inflammation,itching), Nat m, Sep, Staph, Lyco, Apis, Ambra

Syphilis: Merc d, Colotropis g, Merc s, Nit ac, Kreos, Aur mur nat, Syphilinum 1M.

PREGNANCY AND LABOR

Agalactia (Mother after child birth): Puls(milk absent), Utr u(arrest flow of milk), Ricinus com(Increase the quantity of milk), Lac c, Lac d, Bell, Chin(over lactation), Asaf, Agn.

Anemia of pregnancy: Calc p, Ferr m, Ferr p.

Child bed fever: Acon, Bapt, Bry, Arn, Ars, Echin, Kali p, Lach, Merc c, Merc s(milk fever), Acon, Bry, Calc, Cham (high septic fever)

Decline after child birth: Acet ac, Calc p, Carbo an, Carbo v, Caust, China, China s, Kali c, Nat m, Phos ac.

Delayed labour: Bell, Chamom, Gelsi, Puls, Scale c.

Falls Labor pains: Coulophy, Cimicifuga, Puls.

Glactorrhoea (Excessive flow of milk in breasts): Asaf,Bell, Bry, Calc c, Cham, Con, Lact c, Lact v, Medusa, Phos, Phyt, Sabal,

Lochia (slow bleeding from womb after birth): Arn, China, Ipec, Millef, Sabina, Trill,Crocus

Intermittent flow: Graph, Puls, Kreos

In prolonged: Caul, Cham, Ham, Kreos, Nit ac, Pyrog, Sec.

Dark red lochia: Caul, Cham, Ham, Kreos, Nit ac, Pyrog, Sec.

Lochia worse from motion: Erig, Litt, Millef, Sec, Trill.

Mastitis: (Inflamation of breasts): Bell, Boarx, Bry, Calc c, Phyto (pain), Puls.

Milk fever: Bry

Morning sickness: Aletris f, Anac, Carbolium ac, Ipec, Kresoso, Nat p, Nux v, Sep.

Pain less Delivery: Acon, Arn, Couloph, Gelsi, Phos, Sil, Staphsagria.

Pre mature Delivery: Acon, China, Phos, Puls.

Pregnancy of hysterical: Act rac

Pregnancy bleeding (3rd month): Sacle,Sabina, Corc s, Kreost

Pregnancy bleeding (5th-7th month) : Sepia

Pregnancy in piles: Collin,Capsi

Pregnancy in toothache: Merc c

Pregnancy in constipation: Sepia

Pregnancy in after delivery breast swollen; Puls

Prolonged or difficult labour: Arn, Chamm, Coffe, Gelsi, Plum m.

Pregnancy complaints after delivery: Lachesis

Prevention of Abortion: Coulophyllum, Cimici, Ferr p, Merc s, Phos, Sabina, Sepia.

PRAGNANCY DISORDERS

Albuminuria: Apis

Aversion of food: Laur

Backache: Kali c, Sars

Blindness: Ranculus bulbosus

Breast pain: Con, Sep

Burning anus: Capsi

Constipation: Sep

Constant Hacking cough: Kali bi

Cramps: Varat a

Desire un unusual articles of food: Chelli

Diarrhoea: Puls, Nux v, Cham, Phos ac.

Digesty troubles: Calc f

Foetus displacement: Puls

Great falling hair: Sep, Nat m

Heart burn/acidity: Calc c, Puls, Lyco

Labour like pains: Caulo

Oedema of legs: Bry, Sulf

Salivation: Merc sol

Sleeplessness: Anca

Swelling of feet and face: Apis

Septic fever in after delivery: Phyrogenium

Uren expelled (Bladder): Caust 4 hourly

Utters bleeding after delivery: Pituta

Varicose veins: Puls,Lach,Nux

Vomiting: Colch, Sep

Weakness in lower limbs: Agar

RESPIRATORY TROUBLES

Asthma: Acon,Ars,Anti tart, All sat, Alli urs,Baccili, Blatta ori, Carbo v, Dros, Eucal, Hydroc ac, Hep, Ipec, Kali c, Lob inf, Nat s, Nux v,Med, Passi flo, Samb, Syph,Viscum, Tuber.

Asthma cardiac: Acon, Adon v, Ars, Ars iod, Bry, CactQ +Cart Q IN 1:3 Ratio,Carb v, Ipec, Sumbul, Stoph, Lberis. Grinda,

Asthma children: Thuj, Psorinum

Asthma of old persons: Ambra, Bry, Ipec, Asaf, Carb v, Ars (12 in night), Baccillinum, Nat s, Anti c, Arg n, Apis,Stram, Cupram, Lobe inf, Cham, Hep,

Asthma chronic: Hep

Bronchitis: prevents – Calc c, Sul, Phos.

Bry, Kali bi, Puls, Am c, Naphaline, Dros, Anti iod, Phos, Bacill, (Children – Fer p, Infants- Ipec, Anti t.

Burning heat in chest: Acon, Am c, Am m, Apis, Ars, Bell, Brom, Bry, Calc c, Carb v, Cic, Kreos, Lyco, Mag m, Merc, Phos, Sang, Sang n, Spong, Sul, Wyeth.

Chest pain: Acon, Am m, Arn, Asclep, Ars, Bell, Bry, Cact, Calc c, Carb v, China, Cim, Caust,Gauic, Kali c, Lob inf, Mag p, Nat s, Eup perf, Ran b, Rumex, , Sang, Sticta, Sul, Ther.

Cold, Cough and Coryza with flu or influenza: Acon, Ars, Ars iod, Bapt, Bell, Brom, Bry, Carb ac, Cepa, China, China s, Dulc, Eucal, Ering, Eup perf, Euph, Gels,Influz, Nat s, Nux v, Rhus t, Rumex, Sabad, Sag.

Cough cardic: Hydrocyanic ac, Dig, Naja, Lauroucerasus, Capsi.

Cough dry: Bell

Emphysema (destruction of air passage of the lungs): Anti t, Aspidosper, Bry, Carb v, Coca, Napthalinum, Senega, Strachinum pur.

Esophagus: Acon, Bell, Naja, Alumina, Bapti, Phos, Amm c, Asfoeteda, Caust, Canth, Phos(burning),Bryt c, Coculus ind, Crotalus.

Hoarseness sore throat: Phos, Arum t

Hoarseness catarrhal with expectoration of mucus: allium cepa

Hoarseness damp air: Carb v

Hoarseness sudden: Arum t

Hoarseness weakness of vocal card: Rhus tox

Laryngitis (Inflammation, pain worse talking): Phos

Pleurisy: Acon, Hep, Ars, Chin, Canth, Abrot, Hip ac (Right), Bry

Pneumonia: Bry, Anti t 1M, Kali s, Hep, Vert v, Acon,Ferru p, Ars, Kali m.

Broncho Pneumonia: Ars,Ars iod, Anti t, Bry, Cheli, Ipcc, Iod, Lyco, Phos, Sang, Sul.

CIRCULATORY DISEASES

Action of heart intermittent and week (Body weekness, Anemic look, week action of heart, Dizzeness, Sluggish circulation,Dullness of head, heavy numb cold etc...): Acon, Adon v, Am m, Apocy, Ars, Cact,Cart, Carb v, Calc p, Con v, Dig, Gels, Hydroc, Kal, Luplu, Lycop, Nat m, Mur ac, Acid phos, Sep, Spig, Stroph, Verat v.

Action of heart fast and violent: Abies, Acon, Agar, Bell, Cact, Cart, Carb v, Conv,Glon, Kal, Lycop, Nat m, Naja, Nux M, Nux v, Mosch, Physost, Puls, Spig, Spong, Stroph, Iod,Verat v.

Angina pectoris (constructing pains around heart): Mag p, Cmic, Act rac, Cactus g, Carta, Ars iod 3x, Cup ac, Lactrodectus mactons, Glon, Spig, Bry, Ergot.

Arterio sclerosis (walls are thickness): Bar m, Kali p, Visc, Arn, Plb, Adren, Aur m, Ergotam, Nat I, Strophanthus, and CardusQ.

High BP: Aur m, Bar m, Bell, Cart, Glon, Biscum, Lach, Nat m, Sang, Kli p, Rauwolfia, Bar c, Visc, Adren, Pic ac(Kidneys), Gels.

Low BP: Acon, Apis, Gels, Acetanilidum, Chin, Carb v, Camph, Lycpus, Nat m, Nux v, Sep, Verat a, Viscm.

Dropsy: Apis, Adon v, Apocy, Arn, Ars, Cact, Conv, Collins, Caffeine, Crat Digi, Iod, Laitris, Lycop, Stroph.

Endocarditis (inflammation of the living membrane of the heart): Acon, Ars alb, Digiti, Naja, Termila arjuna.

Heart enlargement: Aon, Adon v, Arn, Ars,Am c, Ars, Bar c, CactQ + Crat Q (1:3), Cim, Conv, Digi, Gels, Iberis, Lycop, Naja, Physost, Spart s, Spig, Stroph.

Heart fluttering / Gastric: Abies n, Acon, Arg n, Ars, Bry, Cact Q+ CratQ(1:3), Carb v, Calc p, Camph, China, Coca, Coff, Gent, Ipec, Lyco, Lob inf, Nux v, Puls, Verat a.

Pain around in the heart: Acon, Anac, Ars iod, Arg n, Bry Q, Cact Q+ CratQ(1:3), Carb v, Gent, Ipec, Lyco, Lycop, Lob inf,Nat m, Nux v, Puls, Spig.

Endocarditic: Aon, Adon v, Apis, Ars iod,, Bry, Bell, Bar c, CactQ + Crat Q (1:3), China s, Colch, Conv, Digi, Kali c, Kali iod, Aur iod, Kal, Lach, Merc s, Naja, Nat m, Spig, Spong, Sul, Verat a.

 Varicose veins (fore head, neck, chest, legs): Alum, Ambra, Anti t, Arn, Arg n, Ars, Bell, Calc c, Calc f, Carb an, Carb v, Calc iod, Card m, Flour ac, Graph, Ham, Lycopus, Nat m, Paeonia, P[lum,Puls, Staph, Sul, Vipera.

Varicose Ulcer: Carb v,Hamam.Hyper,Laches,Pul

<u>BODY BACK AND EXTREMITIES</u>

Anemia- spinal (Great weekness, debility, heaviness, numbness, soreness of spinal or back bone patient feel pain in back bone ,worse by pressing, working, walking, ascending steps and by exertion): Aesc, Agar, Alumen, Alum, Alum sil, Ars n, Ars, Aur mur, Berb v, Calc p, China, Cin, Cocc, Con, Ferr m, Ferr p, irid, Kali p, Nat m, Phos ac, Plumb m, Plumb iod, Ox ac, Sec, Sel, SDil, Strych p, Tar h, Zinc m.

Ankle Sprained (swelling and pain worse by motion or by touching the ground): Am, Carbo an, Led, Nat c, Ruta.

Ankle weakness: Nat m, Sil, Calc c, Calc p.

Arthritis: Act sp, Bry, Caust, Colch (swelling of knees) , Dul, Kalm, Merc s, Rhus t, Sil, Sul

Arthritis chronic: Arbut, Bry, Colch, Guaiac, Led, Lyco, Med, Puls, Sul. Stic (right shoulder), Sal ac (joint selling, redness and high fever), Pic ac, Seng, Ruta, Puls, Rhus t, Calc, Hyp, Phos, Nat p, Cadmium, Thuja(gonorrhea).

Atrophy of nipples and breast: Sarsaparilla, Nux m, Con.

Backache: Berb v, Nux v, Aesculus, Tellu, Ant t, Variolinum

Back aching due to different causes: Arn (over exertion), Kali c (pregnant women), Ter (scanty urine), Ox ac (Oxalates in urine), Aesc (piles), Verat v (Small pox), Cimici f. Rhus t, Calc c, Gnapha, Puls (menstruation), Agar (stiff spine), Act rac, Sec cor.

Blistering (in flamed boils on face, fingers, hands and legs): Anac, Anti c, Apis, Ars, Borax, Bry, Buro, Canth, Carbo an, Carbo s, Caust, Cham, Clem, Dulc, Graph, Hep, Kali ars, Kali c, Mag c, Merc, Nat s, Nat m, Nat p, Ran b, Rhus t, Sec, Sep,Sil, Sul.

Bone ache: Amm c, Eup perf,

Bone abnormal growth and swelling: Merc c, Rhus t, Kali I, Calc f, Calc p

Bone (ricket, and diseases of hip joint): Sili, Calc c

Bone enlargement: Calc f

Bone fracture: Calc, Symphtum 1M, Ruta g

Bone inflammation: Ruta, Symphy, Hecla lava,

Bone pains (fracture or injury): Asaf, Ruta

Bones swelling of fingers and knees: Cochi

Burning: Acon, Agar, Apis, Avena, Bry, Calc c, Calc s, Canth, Carb v, Cham, Graph, Lach, Lyco, Med, Puls, Sang, Sul, Sanic.

Burning Feets: Arundo, Calc c, Calc s, Cantha, Hyperi, Lyco, Meddor, Sanguria, Sanicula, Chemomilla, Sul (night).

Burning Hands: Apis, Canth, Utrica u, Arn, Bell, Calendula oint, Caust, Hep sul, Hyper, Phos.

Buttocks: Acid p, Bellis, Calc p. Graph, Gauic, Kalium c, Lythyrus, Rhus t, Stapha,.

Caries (Long bones and their tissues and skulls): Acid fl, Asfoetida, Aur m, Brayt c, Calc c, Sil, Calc fl, Calc p, Coca, Theridion, Con, Heckla, Hepr, Kresostum, Phos, Staph, Strontium nit.

Cholesterol: Allium sat, Avena sat, Chrysanth, Crataegus oxy, Embelica, Ginseng, Guggul, Lecith, Lyco, Oenoth, Sugar cane wax, Terminalia arj, Balerica.

Chilblains: Agar, Puls, Acid n, Tamus communis.

Clairvoyance: Aconit, Agaricus mus, Iodium.

Claustrophobia: Arg nit, Succinum.

Clumsiness (numbness of hands & fingers): Apis, Bovista.

Coccyx (last bone in the spine): Ant t, Bovista, Carb an, Castor equi, Casti, Arn, Ruta, Cicuta v, Euphorbinum o,Hypericum, Kali bich, Laches, Paeonia, Platin m, Sil, Xanthum.

Coldness of back and numbness of limbs: Abies, Acon, Agar, Arg m, Ambra, Arg n, Ars, Bell, Benz ac, Calc c, Calc p, CactQ+ CartQ(1:3), Carb v, Chaina, Cocca, Con, Dig, Dul, Gels, Helon, Hydro c ac, Lyco, Nux m, Nat m, Onosm, Phyto, Pic ac, Plat, Raph, Sil, Sep, Strych, Thall, Verat a, Zin m.

Collapse: Camphora Q, Carb v, Cup m, Glonium, Hydrocynum ac, Srontim c, Vetram alb.

Coma: Alluminum m, Amm c, Amylenum nit, Arn, Asafoetida, Sep, Baptisia, Bryt c, Camphora, Gelsi, Helleborus, Hep sul, Lach, Mosch, Nux m, Opium, Renuneculs b, Verat alb.

Complexion: Berberi aq, Iod, Sarasaparilla.

Corns: Acid p(painful), Anti crud, Ferr pic, Radium brom, Graph(corn & cracks), Hydrastis, Nit ac, Selen, Sul, Verat vir, Thuja, Wiesbaden.

Cracks: Calc fl, Cistus, Graph, Nat m, Nit acid, Petro, Sarasa, Tamus.

Cracking of joints: Amm m, Benz ac, Bry, Caust, Cimex, Colo, Cocc,Diosc, Graph, Med, Nat ars, Nat m, Nux v, Ruta, Sul.

Carmps: Verat a, Sul, Colo, Ferr m, Scrophul, Vib o, Cholos terrapinoe, Cupram, Asaf (Hysterical patient)

Edema (swelling): Acetic ac, Anti ars, Anti tart, Apis, Apocy, Ars alb, Aur m, Bry, Cactus, Hydrocoty, Kali carb, Phos, Rhus t, Sanguri, Tarentula, Terbenth, Thyrodi, Vesicara.

Elephantiasis: Calotro, Hydrocoty, Myristic seb.

Exertion (stamina): Sterculia a,Coca

Feet burning: Arundo, Calc c, Calc sul, Cantha, Hyperi, Lycopo (at night), Medorr, Sanguia, Sanicula, Sulph.

Feet cool: Acon, Bryt c, Bell, Calc c, Campho, Colchi, Nat p, Pic ac, Scale c, Sili,

Feet sweaty: Arundo, Calc c, Carb v, Iodium, Lyco, Sili.

Feet pains: Colotropis, Chamomilla, Eupt perf, Halonius, Ledum, Lithium c, Medorr,

Fingers rhumatism: Agricus m, Anti c, Apis, Arg m, Beri beri v, Borax, Cauloph, Cina, Graph, Hyperi, Ledum, Nat m, Petrol, Rhus t, Sarasap, Sili, Thuja.

Gout: Benz ac, Lith c, Led, Pic ac, Rhododen, Berb v, Colchi, Sars, Acid p (long bones), Staph (all joints), Chin, Cupram ac(swollen joints), Aesc (neuralgic), Asaf (nervous), Colchi (toe and heal).Utri u (joint pain), Abrot(joint stiff), Bell (swelling),

Hands: Acon & Calend (cold), Apis (swellon), Calc c(sweating), Caust(no sensation), Colchicum (jerking), Phos(burning), Ranunculus (itching), Sarasapa(craks),

Hands Pain: Apis, Mel

Heel Pain: Agar, Am c, Am m, Arn, Berb v, Caps, Ign, Caust, Colchi, Graph, Led, Nit ac, Phos ac, Phyto, Puls, Rhus t, Ruta, Sabina, Sep, Sil, Thuj, Valer, Zinc.

Hip joint pain: Ars, Arg m, Berb v, Bry, Calc c, Calc p, Caust, Chel, Cistus, Colchi, Colo, Con, Gels, Hyper, Kali I, Nat m, Lit t, Stram,Thuja.

Hemophilia: Calc lact, Fucus ind, Hamamel, Laches, Crotolus, Phos, Syzygium.

Hypothermia (immediate increase body temperature): CamphoraQ

Joints Pain with Swelling: Arg m, Bry, Calc p, Caust, Cim, Colch, Gauic, Kalm, Merc s, Lyco, Puls, Rhust, Ruta, Sab, Sul.

Joints Burning: Apis, Ars alb, Caust, Rhus t, Sul.

Joints cracking: Ginseng, Acon

Knee pain: Diosco, Berb v (stiffness, swelling,), Sul, Calc, Taxus, Puls, Cocc, Kali c, Lathyrus sativas.

Legs: Agricus, Alumina, Arn, Bell, Bellis, Calc c, Platinum m (sleep legs), China (pain), Conium (sudden loss of strength), Lyco(jerking), Medorr(legs heavy), Tarentula(numbeness), Zinc m.

Leukemia: Ars iod, Ars hydr, Bryt mur, Benzium, Calc c, Calc fl, Calc p, Ceanothus, China of, Chinunum sul, Ferr pic, Merc sol, Calc c, Nat sul, Psori, Radium brom, Thiosi, Vanadium.

Lice: Lyco, Psori, Staph,

Lips: Aloes, Amm c, Apis, Ars alb, Arum trip, By, Capsicum, Cannabis ind, Conium, Hydrastis, Condrogo, Heper sul. Merc sol, Nat c, Sepia, Nat m, Nux m, Petro, Puls, Sili, Sulph, Tarent.

Lumbago: Agar, Berb v, Bell, Belli p, Gnaph, Cimc f, Aloes, Calc p, Nux v, Aesculus, Tellu, Ant t, Kali c, Kali p, Led, Lac c, Mag c, Rhus t, Symph, Variolinum, Zinc

Loco motor (loss of sensitivity in lower limbs): Gels, Arg n, Phos, Alumina, Apis, Angustura, Sec, Agar.

Moles (birth marks): Acid fl, Bellis (external), Calc c, Lyco, Radium brom. Thuja.

Muscular pain: Rhus t, Plumb, Caust 1m, Carb an, Agar (jerking), Arn, Hyos, Acon, Ambar.

Nail pain: Ber v

Nails blue, falling, pain: Qxalic ac, Hellebours f(falling), Thuja (soft nails), Sep (pains), Stanm (spilting).

Nails biting: Aurum trip, Ambr, Sanic, Amm bro (nervous irritation)

Nail color spots: Sil (White), Am c (yellow), Ars (Blue)

Nails diseases: Amm brom, Amm c, Anti c, Beri beri vulg, Hellebrous, Hypericum, Nat m, Nit ac, Oxalicum ac, Sarasapa, Sepia, Sili, Stramonium, Thuja Webseden.

 Nails finger hurt: Hyperc

Nails fungus: Sepia, Myristica, Calendula.

Nail mis shaped: Acid fl, Calc c, Graph, Thuja

Nail psoriasis: Chyrsophantic ac

Nail skin cracking: Nat m

Neck : Arum t (discharge from nose), Baccili, Sil. Brayt c, Calend (neck enlarged gland), Rhus t (neck sprin), Merc sol (swelling), Acon every hour (neck stiff).

 Neck pain: Acon, Bell, Bry, Caust, Dul, Cim, Gels, Gauic, Mag p, Rhus t,

Osteoporosis: Calc c, Calc p, Cimicifuga, Ginsing, Ginkgo, Sili, Symphytum.

Pains in electrical shock: Acid fl, Cimicifu, Colchic, Phytolacca de.

Pains in Numbness: Acon, Chamomi,Kalium lat, Plati m, Rhus t, Calc p, Kalium c, caust.

Pains in sensitive parts: Acon, Chamomi, Coffe c.

Pains in sensation of fullness: Assculs hip, China, Lyco.

Pains in Neurotic: Agricus m

Pains in bons: Amm c, Eup perf, Aurm m, Kali bich, Asafoetida, Merc sol.

Pains inbones of extremities and heels: Aranea diad, Bellis, Eup perf, Ruta.

Pains are burning: Ars a, Bell, Canth, Capsic, Phos, Sul.

Pains relived by warmth: Ars a, Apis.

Pains in bone: aur m.

Pains in changed : Beri beri vulg.

Pains better by rest : Bry

Pains are cutting and stitching: Bry, Kali c,

Pains in sore and bruised: Arnica, Bapt, Pyroge.

Pains in chest: Calc c

Pains with sensation of coldness: Camph, Secal c, Heloderma, Puls, Calc c, Ars, Cistus, Verat alb.

Pain in right sholder/right elbow: Ferrum mur, Phytolacca d.

Pains in walking and sitting: Gnaphili.

Pains after operation: Hyperic.

Pains in limbs: Indigo

Pains in pressure: Kali c, Colocynth, Rhus t, Sepi, Mag p.

Pains in hifting wendering: Kali sul.

Pains in Nerualgic: Kalima lat

Pains in any were: Lachesis

Pancreas inflamation: Arg nit,Chinothus,Merc sol, Bell, Kali iod.

Pancreas (stone): Fragaria vesca

Pancreas (cancer): Iodium

Pancreas (Fatty): Phos

Pancreas(gastric/ vomting/ nausea/indigestion): Iris vers, Pepsium

Paralysis: Arg n (memory), Caust & Coni (eyes due to exposure), Coni & Zinc m and Brat c (neuralgia), Opium (stool, bladder, urination), Caust (eye lid right side), Alumn (rectal inertia & constipation), Senega (left side face), Caust (right side of face), Gelsi, Coni, Acon, Plb (hands), Cimic, Agar. Lach (vocal card).

Rheumatic pain: Apis, Ac benz, Bry, Caul, Caust, Cim, Colch, Gauic, Kali iod, Kalm, Lac c, Led, Lith c, Merc s, Phos ac, Phyto, Puls, Rhus t, Sul, Verat v.

Sacrum: Laches, Sabina, Sepi, Tellurium m, Aesculus, Aloes, Bapti, Beriberi v, Helonias

Sciatica: Medorrhinum (chronic), Kali b, Bry, Rut, Caust, (left side), Colchi, Phyt, Nux v, Carb s, Gnaphi, Cotyledon tin, Lyco, Tell, Hyperi, Phytos, Iodum, Apocy (Odema), Rhus t, Gnaphi, Lyco, Disco, Kali p, Mag p (right side), Acid s, Coloc, Viscum, Cimici f(lumbgo).

Scapula: Amm m, Bryt c & Rhus t (sholder blades), Chelido & Chenopodium (right sholder), Sulphar (left sholder).

Sholder pains: Kreost & Caust (left), Chenapodi, Rhus t, Podophy, Sangui,Ferr m (right).

Slipped disc: AScon, Amm c, Apis, Arn, Bell, Bry, Caust, Hyper, Kaliu bich, Kali c, Ledu, Nux v, Rhus t.

Snoring: China, Hippozaeninum, Lemna minor, Oenanthe croc, Opium.

Speech: Bryt m(talks nose), Cannabis s(defects of speech), Hyper(jerking), Laches(stiuffness of tongue), Agriphus nut(child hood not speak).

Spleen: Caloc ars & Ceanothus and China, Ferr arsm Ferr iod(enlarge), Fragaria vesca(stone), Laches(pain),

Spondylitis: Acid p, Cocculus ind, Dulc, Kalium iod, Mag p, Calc flour, Kali m, Theridion.

Stamina: Coca, Sterculia aq,Zinc p.

Steroids: Bryt iod, Calc p, Cheli, Hyoscy, Oopho,Orchiti,

Sternum: Aur met, Caust, Merc sol, Taraxcum.

Stiffness of body: Abrot, Acon, Agar, Am m, Arg n, Berb v, Calc c, Calc p, Caust, Cim, Cocc, Con, Cup ars, Dul, Ginsing, Helon, Kail c, Kali p, Led, Lyco, Phyto, Gauic, Rhus t, Ruta, Sep, Sil, Strych, Sul.

Sweating of axillae, hands and feet: Am m, Bart c, Bov, Calc c, Carb v, Cocc, Con, Flour ac, Graph, Her, Kail c, Lyco, Nat m, Nit ac, Osmium, Petrol, Picr ac, Psori, Rhus t, Sep, Sil, Sul, Strych p, Tellur, Thuja, Wyteth

Sweating Hands: Sulph, Calc c, Sil,Lyco, Ign.

Sweating Feet: Psori, Sulph, Merc sol, Calc c, Sili, Graph.

Wrists (rheumatism): Caulophy, Euip perf, Kalium c, Mag p, Nat p, Trimethylaminum.

SKIN DISEASES

Abscess : Bell, Apis, Hep, Arn, Calc s, Fl ac, Sang, Ars, Tarent, Anthra, Sil,Rhus t, Echni, Pyroge, Kali iod, Lach, Vespa, Carb ac, Merc sol, capsicum,

Acne (Pimples): Asterias rubens, Kali b, Radium bro, Ars I, Sul I, Hydrc, Hep sul, Led,Nit ac, Bor, Hep, Ant t, Kali br, Aur and Dros (black pores), Jugl c, Psori, Petrol, Nux v, Nat m, Led,Sil.

Allergy (sudden swelling, puffing, reddening, burning, and itching)/ cold: Apis (heat), Ars alb (cold), Choloratum (alcoholic), Dulcmara (damp whether), Utrica ur, Nat p, Nat sul, Sul, Canth, Graph, Arg nit, Nat m, Camphor & Nux v (allopath medicines),

Allergy in food: Onion – Thuja, Sugar – Sacch, Eggs and Animal cooking food – Lecithin & Feer m and Tub, Fish – Ferr m, Wheat – Psori, Milk products – Tub & Sul, Colthing – Cort c, Oils – Puls, Milk – Nat c, Water – Sel, Beer – Leach.

Alopecia: Acid f, Aloe, Bryt c, Cantha, Sili, Vinc m, Baccili, Tub, Thuja.

Blisters: Allu c (Nails), Nat m & Ign (Mouth / Fever), Thuja, Phos acid, Apis, Bapti (with fever), Canth (with burns), Mag mur, Medorrh, Hyper.

Blotches: Primula obconia

Boils: Lyco, Pic ac (ear), Berb (anus with fistula), Echi Q, Hyper, Am c, Carbo ani, Sul, Arn, Thuja, Bry, Luet, Anthar & Ars a, Terent c and Lach (carbuncles), Sep (childerns), Hepr s or Calc s (discharges), Tuber (nose), Bell Ternt c(Swelling).

Burning: Caust, Urt u, Canth, Hyper (anti septic), Calend, Capsi, Carbic ac, Ambra, Kali bich.

Carbucle: Ars, Lach, Anthra, Am c, Myris, Abroma a, Apis, Tarent, Bell.

Chicken Pox: Rhust, Anti c, Bry, Thuja, Vario, Anti t, Achyranthes calea (Cow pox / Chicken pox/Measles), Sarr.

Chilblains/ crackes: Acid n, Rhus t, Tam, Abrot, Aur, Agar, Petr. Puls,

Cicatrix / scar:

Dandruf: Badiga, Lac c, Thuj, Phos, Ars, Kali bi, Vinc, Nat m, Graph, Lyc.

Dermatitis: Bell, Sil, Apis, Spong, Sars, Rhus t, Graph, Achyranthes calea, Arn.

Eczema: Anac, Agar, Cic, Graph, Kali br, Skookam c, Tub, Tell, Vinc. **Eczema all over body** – Bacc, Tub, Syphi, **Eczema of diabetis** – Dol, **Eczema of blood purified** – Gunp, Sarasapa, **Eczema of anckles** – Selini, **Eczema of anus** – Graph, **Eczema of gouty persons-** Led, **Eczema of hair** – Sulph,Nat m, Calc c, **Eczema in flod of neck-** Hydrast, **Eczema in genitals-** Corton, **Eczema pustular-** Clem, **Eczema red blotches** – Fragopyrum, **Eczema in sclap** – Psori, Cicuta, **Eczema with swelling glands** – Tub, Syphl, Anti t, Hama, Echin, Hydrast, Anac, Juglan, Kali ars, **Eczema blister-** Rhus t, **Eczema ears-** Lyco, Graph, **Eczema on face-** Kali m, **Eczema on hands / fingers -** Mezer, Graph, Bovista, Carb v, Merc s, Sulph, Sep, **Eczema of head-** Arum t, **Eczema on lid-** Graph, Staph, **Eczema on nose/ lips-** Alum, Kali c, Phos, **Eczema wet-** Sep, Graph, **Eczema and other skin trobles-** Calc, **Eczema of vescular-** Kali s, **Eczema sclap-** Agar, Rhust t, Cicuta, **Eczema itching** – Anac, Streptoccon, **Eczema of long duration-** Auram m, Merc s, Kali chlor, **Eczema drugs for external use -** AlunsQ, Adrenalin chlor, Bicorborate soda with worm wter.

Eczema Dry: Alumina, Calc sul, Chrysa, Sul, Tuber.

Eruption: Lyco, Jug c, Bry, Sulph, Varioli, Petr, Astac, Olender, Cort t, Rhust, Thuj, Nat m, Aurum t, Am c, Sil, Ant t, Anac,

Erysipelas: Bell, Caust,Anthra, Aconi. Apis, Graph, Lach, Passi, Rhust t.

Erythema: Acon, Apis, Atipyr, Arn, Bell, Canth, Cham, Fagop, Graph, Lyco, Merc s, Petrol, Puls, Rhust t.

Fissures: Graph, Petr, Thuj, Merc, Paeon, Lac d, Nat m, Am c, Nit ac, Platina, Rat, Led, Calendula, Crocus.

Fistula: Hydra, Nit ac, Sil, Bacilli, Berb v, Thuj, Bell, Merc s, Calc f, Sulf, Aesc, Caust, Chin, Rat, Phos. **Fistula anus-** Merc, Graph, Cal, Sil, Calend, **Fistula Root of teeth-** Fl ac, **Fistula of the glands-** Phos, Sil, Merc, **Fistula of eyes** – Sulph, Puls, Hyper s, ,Calend lotion, Fistula with piles – Sil, **Fistula of vagina** – Puls, Asa c, Nit ac, Petrs,Thuj, Lach, Anti.

Freckle (brown spot on skin / sun burn): Am c, Ant t, Bry, Calc, Dulc, Ferr, Graph, Lyco, Mur ac, Nat c, Nit ac, Phos, Puls, Sep, Sul.

Fungal diseases: Alumen, Ars alb, Borax, Calc c, Echina, Laches, Lyco, Manicula, Phos, Sep, Sili, Thuja.

Gangreen: Ars, Anthar, Bell, Acet ac, Carb v, Crotalus, Echin, Lach, Secle cor, Sulph ac. Sec.

Gonorrhea: Agnus c, Arg nit, Copaiva, Kreoso, Merc c, Nat sul, Sili, Thuja.

Herpes: Ars, Ambr, Alumina, Anthra, Agar, Calo,Crotal h, Dol, Iris, Merc, Mezer, Ran b, Rhust t, Sulo ac.

Hives: Ant c, Anthrak, Apis, Ars, Bov, Calc c, Chliral, Cop, Cort t, Dul, Kali c, Lyco, Nat p, Puls, Rhus t, S   ul, Utr u.

Ignoring toe nails: Ant c , Caust, Flour ac, Graph, Hep, Nit ac, Sil, Staph, Thuj.

Impertigo (inflammatory skin): Ant c, Ant t, Ars, Cic, Clem, Dulc, Graph, Hep, Kali bi, Lyco, Mez, Rhus t, Sep, Sil, Sul, Thuj, Viola.

Injuries: Arn, Bellis, Calend, Calc p, Hyper, Conium, Led, Hep, Millef, Ruta, Sul ac.

Insect bites: Acet ac (cat bite), Apis (sting bites), Utr u, Lach, Golondrina (Snake Poison), Led (cat, dog, rat etc..), Caust, Cedr (Anti dot in snake poison),Hydroph (dog), Naja (snake).

Itching: Abrot, Agar, Ambr, Alumi, Antimonium sul & Bryt c (old people), Crot t, Heper, Hydrocoti, Merc, Olender, Psori, Ran b, Seline(joints), Sulph, Sul ac.

Itching Dry: Alum, Anac, Ars, Aur mur, Berb aq, Bov, Bry, Calc p, Clem, Bar c, Cham, China, Dolich, Dulc, Eup perf, Gels, Graph, Lach, Med, Merc, Mez, Petr, Led, Kali ars, Kali c, Lyco, Nux m, Plumb, Psori, Sec, Sars, Serl, Sep, Sul.

Keloid: Acid fl, Graph, Sili, Thiosi, Tuberc.

Lecoderma: Ars sul, Hydrocot, Tuber, Nit ac (white spot), Ars (white skin), Psoral, Nat m, Bacc.

Leprosy: All-s, Ars, Anac, Bacc, Colotropis, Chalimugra, Hydroc, Hura brasiliensis.cm, Huyang nak.

Measles: Acon, Achyranthes calea, Ars, Bry, Bell, Euphra, Ferr p, Hydrast, Kali bich (respiratory symptom), Kali m, Puls, Rhust t, Sil, Stram, Vario.Vert a. **Measles restlessness** - Puls, Rhust t.

Measles restlessness – Sulph, Merc s, Nat m, Puls. **Measles prophylactics** – Acon, Ars, Morbillinu, Puls.

Naevus: Acet ac, Calc c, Carb v, Flour ac, Graph, Lyco, Nit ac, Puls, Thuj.

Needle stiching: Acon, Apis, Bry, Mag p, Nat m, Nat p, Nat s, Puls, Ranb, Rhumex, Sul,

Nodous or knotty skin: Ant c, Dulc, Graph, Calc c, Calc fl, Led, Lyco, Ran b, Rhus t, Sep, Sul, Thuj.

Pimples: Ambra, Adren, Arn, Aurum , Acon, Abroma, Berb aq, Bell, Elec, Lac d.

Pruritus: Acon Am c, Ambr, Aeth, Alum, Dol, Dulc, Calad, Iod, Sul.

Psoriasis: Ars, Ars br, Adren, Borax, Caps, Cupr, Graph, Hep, Iod, Kali s, Lyc, Med, Merc, Nit ac, Psori, Petr, Rad br, Rhust t, Sul, Thyr, Thuj.

Rashes: Acon, Am c, Ant t, Ars, Bell, Con, Ipec, Rhust t, Thuja.

Ring worm: Ant c, Ars, Bry c, Bry c, Calc c, Cort t, Graph, Hep, Kali s, Lyco, Mez, Petr, Rhust, Sep, Staph, Tell, Sul, Dul (Hair), Hell & Tell (face and chest), **Ring worm on sclap of children in face, neck, eyes-** Rhus, Sul, Staph, Heper.

Scurvy (lack of vitamin c): Merc, Dulc, Carb v, Lach, Acet ac, Abies n, Ferr p.

Skin: Sep (brown spot), Sanic (skin flabby), Abrot & Rad br (all skin problems), Lac d (cold skin/swetting), Sul (dirty skin), Thuj (yong acne face).

Small Pox: Ars, Acon, Arn, Ant t, Acet ac, Maladrenum, Serr, Vac, Variolinum, Thuj.

Skin Thick: Agar, Alum, Anac, Ars, Ars iod, Bryt c, Bor, Calc c, Carb an, Cort t, Con, Dulc, Graph, Hydrocot, Iod, Lach, Lith, Lyco, Led, Mang, Merc, Mur ac, Petr, Ran b, Rhus t, Sec, Sep, Sil, Sul Nat c, Nat m, Plumb, Thuj.

Skin wrinkled: Ambr, Anti c, Ars, Bor, Con, Cupr, Kali ars, Kreos, Lyco, Mez, Phos ac, Phyto, Sars, Sec, Sep, Sul, Verat a, Veart v.

Scabies: Abro Am m, Ars, Hep, Crot t, Lach, Nat m, Psori, Sul, Sil.

Skin Oily: Arg m, Bry, But ac, Calc c, Carbo an, Carbo v, China, Hep-, Lupul, Lyco, Mag c, Merc s, Nit ac, Nux v, Rob, Sel, Sep,Psori, Sil, Staph, Stram, Sumb, Thuj, .

Sopts: Ars a(block), Bell / Berberis aq/ Terent/ Telluri (red spots), Graph & sulph (white), Helliebours & Laches(blue), Nat c& Phos(yellow), Sili(rose), Thuja (brown), Scale cor & Phos (black), Lyco (moles in body),

Sweatting: Ambar, Anthra, Bry, Calc, China, Merc, Petr (feet), Sul, Tell, Thuj, Verat (fore head).

Swollen bites that itch and sting-Utrica uren
Warts: Ambar, Anac, Ant c, Bacc, Caust, Lac c, Lac c, Nat m, Nit ac, Sabin, Thuj.

Wounds: Anthra, Apis, Ars, Acet ac, Arn, Cic, Chin, Hyper, Lach, Led, Sil, Staph, Sympht, Sul ac, Pyrog.

FEVER SYMPTOMS

Chilliness or shivering with fever: Acon, Anti t, Anthra, Ars, Arn, Aur, Bell, Bry, Camph, Gelsi, Sep, Sili, Verat.

Fever: Bell, Bapt, Chin, Chinin s, Cedron, Dul, Ip, Nat m, Pyrog, Thyphoid, Acon (Fever with thirst), Nat m (fever –blisters), **Fever chill with swet-** Calc, **Fever chilly with thirst-**Ignt, **Fever pains /swaet-** China, **Hepitic fever-** Aceat ac, **Fever with cough/ urticaria-** Rhus t, **Sterling child-** Gels, **High fever/burning/no thirst/ feet icy cold/ Delirious condition-** Bell,Acon, Bry,**Fever with smelling stool-** Bapt, **Fever Dentition-** Cham, **eruptive /irregular rash-** Ail,**Swollen and enlarged tonsils-** Bell, Calc, Phyt, Bart c, Calc I, Kali I, Bacill, **Fever influenza-** Ars a, Sul, Gelsi, Eupat perf, Caust, Influeinum, **Malaria-** Rhus t, Nat m, Sul, Cerd, Chinm s, **Milk fever-** Bell, **Fever deafness** – Verat, **Desentry** – Acon, **Rhumatic** – Acon, Bell, Bry, Cham, Calc c, Cim, Colch, China s, Dulc, Nux m, Puls, Rhus t, Sul, Verat v.**Septic** – Ars a, Echi, Rhus t, **Talktive** – Podo, **Fever with vomting** – Bry, **Fever due to vaccination** – Merc s, Hep s, Thuj,

Brain fever (Dengue): Ars, Acon, Bell, Gelsi, Cup m, Helli b, Opium, Eup perf, Rhus t.

Scarlet fever: Amm c, Bell, Rhus t, Streptocrocinum.

Typhoid: Bell, Bapt, Ars a, Gelsi, Sul, Phos (pneumonia),Bapt (Diarrhoea), Acid m (haemorrhage), Absinth(sleeplessness), Cup m (unconsciousness), Acid p (weekness), Carb v, Lyco, Asaf, Ter, Agar (Tympanitis).Secale, Aur t, Rhus t, Lach, Anti c,

SLEEP AND TROUBLES

Sleep aggravation after: Lach, Sleep cat nap type: Nux v, Sel, **Sleep child ganashing teeth-** Bell, **Too much sleep-** Scrophularia nodosa, **Sleepiness** – Cimex, Indol, Ig, Coffe, Daph i, Bry, Ambr, Cimicif, Tabac, Cannabis i, Pssi, Tela ar, **During pregnancy-** Coffe, Bell, Anac, Opium,,**Half open eyes-** Lyco

Night walking: Hyoscy, Kali brom, Kali p, Nat m, Sili.

Walk sleep: Kali p

NERVOUS SYMPTOMS

Depression: Psorin, Act rac, Anac, Aur m(suicidal)

Epiliepsy: Hyscya, Ig, Tancetum, Cupr, Kali br, Glon, Bufo, Nit ac, Cic v, AsinthinumQ, Absinth, Zinc valer, Sili, Amyl nit, **Convulsions** – Agar, Sacch o., **Epilipsy recent**- Kali c, Bell, Opium, Hydrast.

Facial Paralysis: Amm p, Caust, Gelsi, Ign, Plum m, Rhus t

Hysteria: Cannb I,Ambra, Asaf, Castor, Cim, Cocc, Croc, Eup ar, Gels, Ig, Kali p, Mosch, Nux m, Plat, Puls, Pothos, Sep, Stram, Tar b, Val, Zinc m.

Lower motor neuron paralysis (No sensory loss): Acon, Arg nit, Lathyrus, Oxalic ac, Plum m.

Monoplegia (paralysis of lower limbs): Arg n, Caust, Cacu ind, Conium, Cupr m, Gelsi, Nux v, Phos, Plumb m, Rhus t.

Myopathies and motor neuron disease (Weekness of muscles): Abrot, Caust, Gelsi, Lyco, Iod, Nat m.

Nervous exhaustion: Ph ac,

Nervousness: Aqui, Ambr, Acon, Absin, Nat ar, Abies n, Cimic, Agn, Sil, Nux v.

Nervous prostration (Brain fag/Neurasthenia): Ambra, Arg nit, Cocullus, Kali p, Nat mur, Pic ac, Strychinum p, Zinc p.

Nerve injury: Hyper (in all),**Nerve sudden blind** –Sant, **Nervous braek down**- Aur m, **Nervous deafness**- Lach, Naja, **Nervous Diarrhoea** – Gels, **Dyspepsia** - Aeth, **Dyspesia with pain in stomach**- Anac,Colocynth,

Nervous patient: Tela urane, **after infection** – Am c, **No stamina**- Sil, **Headeache** – Asaf, **Sensitive nervous**- China, **Nervous trouble**- Phos.

Neuralgia: Kali i (eye), Bell & Sang (right side pain), Mag p (all pain), Acon & Colchi (face), Spig (left side pain), Colchi & Niccolum sulph(any where in the body), Gels (trmbling of limbs),

Neurasthenia (nervous prostration): Nat m, Kali p, Mephitis, Avena s, Coca, Ph ac, Ig, Cannabis i (general weekness), Agn (sexual excess),

Neruritis: Acon, Hyper, Cimic, Ars, Alliu c, Achyra c, Alloxanum, Carbn s.

Numbness: Acon, Agricus, Ambra, Apis, Arg nit, Asfoteda, Avena s, Brt c, Bufo, Cadmium sul, Calc p, Caust, Caculus ind, Coni, Helonias, KALMIA, Nat m, Phos, Pic ac, Rhus t, Scale cor, Tarentula.

Parkinsonism: Bell, Gelsi, Lachesi, Stromonium.

Paralysis: Agricus mu, Arg nit, Causti, Cup m, Gelsi, Hyoscy n, Mygale las, Mag p, Stramonium, Tarentula, Zin m.

Spasm of glottis (vocal card): Bell (child during sleep), All c (hoarse voice), Naja (voice hearing), Lach, Caust, Ant c (loss of voice), Aurm t, Rhus t, Phos, Gels (voice lost suddenly).

Spasm of muscles: Ars, Bapt, Bell, Belli,. Berb v, Bry, Caust, Cim, Cupr ars, Cupr m, Gels, Guaic, Healon, Kali c, Led, Mag p, Mang, Passiflo, Phyto, Physos, Rhus t, Ruta, Sep, Sul, Upas, Angust, Cic, Cocc, Hydro ac, Hyosc, Hyper, Ipec, Mosch, Nux v, Stram, Veart a, Zinc m.

Stammering (breaks or gaps in the flow of speech): Acon, Arg n, Bell, Bov, Cann I, Cic, Carb s, Caust, Cupr, Euphars, Glon,

Hyosc, Iod, Kali br, Lach, Lyco, Mag c, Mag p, Merc, Nat c, Nat m, Nux v, Phos, Plat, Sec, Sil, Spig, Stram, Sul, Vearty a.

Vitality: Sil, Carb v,

TISSUE TROUBLES

Abscess to treat: Gauic, Hep, Lach, Merc s, Myrist, Phyto, Sil.

Bones brittle and thin (soft): Alum, Ambra, Am c, Calc c, Calc p, Calc fl, Diosc, Flour ac, Graph, Iod, Gauic, Phos.

Death or decay of bony tissue: Angsust, Arg m, Ars, Asaf, Aur m, Calc c, Calc p, Calc fl, Calc sil, Flour ac, Hekla, Hep, Kali bi, Kali I, Med, Merc, Mez, Nit ac, Phos ac, Phos, Sil,Symphyt.

Overgrowth of bones: Arg m, Aur m, Aur m, Calc c, Calc fl, Dulc, Flour ac, Hekla, Kali bi, Kali I, Merc c, Merc s, Mez, Nit ac, Phos, Pulmb ac, Puls, Ruta, Sil,Symphyt.

Bone fracture and help to reunion: Alum, Ambra, Am c, Calc c, Calc p, Calc fl, Diosc, Flour ac, Graph, Iod, Gauic, Phos.

Bone pain: Agar,Arg m, Arn, Asaf, Aur m, Calc c, Calc p, Caps, Caust, Cham, China, Cocc, Con, Cupr, Eupr prf, Flour ac, Hep, Ipec, Kali I, Lyco, Lyss, Merc, Mez, Nit ac, Phos ac, Puls, Rhus t, Ruta, Sabina, Sars, Sep, SilStaph, Sul, Thuj,Symphyt.

Bopnc injury with swelling: Acon, Arn, Calc c, Calc p, Ruta, Sul ac, Sympht,

Bruises: Agar,Arg m, Asaf, Calc c, Cocc, Con, Cupr, Hep, Ig, Ipec, Kali bi, Led, Lith, Mang, Mez, Petro, Phos, Puls, Ruta, Sil, Spig, Veart a.

Cellular (pertaining to skin cells): Apis, Bell, Bry, Hep, Merc s, Myrist, Sil.

Consumptive of phthisical disease (TB)s: All sat, Ant iod, Ars iod, Bac, Calc c (not in old people), Calc iod, Calc p, China ars, Cort h, Hyosc, Iod, Kali c, Carbo an, China s, Gauic, Kali nit,

Lycopus, Cocculus in, Osmium, Phos, Sul, Tuber, Yerba, Sant, Sang, Sil, Spong.

Diarrhoea: Acet ac, Arg nit, Arn, Ars iod, Bapt, Calc , Calcp, China, Calc iod, Sacchar, Coto bark Q, Cupr ars, Iod, Phos ac, Phos, Sil.

Dropsy: Adon v, Apis, Appocy, Ars, Cact, Cart, Chainca, Dig, Helleb, Lyco, Samb can.

Early aging: Ail, Ambr, Arg c, Con, Lyco, Carb v, Helon, Nux m, Nux v, Sel, Urica, Urens Q.

Fistula: Agar, Asaf, Bell, Bry, Calc c, Calc fl, Calc p, Calc s, Caust, Cinnab, Con, Flour ac, Hep, Kali I, Lyco, Merc, Nat m, Petro, Phos, Puls, Sil, Staph, Sul, Thuj.

Gangrenous: Am m, Anthra, Ars iod, Bar c, Bry, Calc c, Calc p, Canth, Carb an, Caust,Cic,Con, Crot h,Dulc,Echin,Fl ac, Graph,Hep, Iod, Kali bi, Kali br, Kali iod,Kali p, Lach, Led,Lyco, Merc, Mez, Mur ac, Nit ac, Petro, Phos, Plb, Sec, Staph, Sul, Sul ac, Thuja, Zinc.

GlandsHardend, swollen, pain: Alumen, Bar c, Bell, Bar m, Brom, Calc c, Calc fl, Calc p, Hep, Iod, Kali bi, Con, Phyto, Sil, Thuja.

Inflammation of Spinal cord: Acon, Arn, Arg n, Ars, Bell, Bellis, Bry, Cic, Gels, Cort h, Lathyr, Merc, Nux v, Oz ac, Pic ac, Plumb, Sec, Strych, Zic p.

Obesity: Am br, Am c, Ant c, Ars, Calc ars, Calc c, Calop, Caps, Col, Fucus, Carb v, Graph, Iodo thyr, Kali br, Kali c, Mag c, Phyto, Phto berr, Sabal, Thyr, Tussil, Np.

Inflammation of bone: Acon, Act sp, Arg m, Asaf, Aur iod, Auram m, Bell, Bry, Calc c, Calc p, Conchiolin, Fl ac, Heckla, Heb

Iod, Kali iod, Lapis, Lac ac, Lyco, Mang, Merc s, Mez,Nat Mur, Nit ac, Phos, Phos ac, Psori, Plumb ac, Puls, Ruta, Sil, Staph, Sul.

Bone marrow: Acon,Arg m, Ars m, Bell, Cham, China s, Cim, Conchiol, Gun [poweder, Nat m, Olend, Plumb, Phos ac, Ruta,

Convertion of cartilage in to bone: Acon, Act sp, Arg m, Asaf, Aur iod, Auram m, Bell, Bry, Calc c, Calc p, Conchiolin, Fl ac, Heckla, Heb Iod, Kali iod, Lapis, Lac ac, Lyco, Mang, Merc s, Mez,Nat Mur, Nit ac, Phos, Phos ac, Psori, Plumb ac, Puls, Ruta, Sil, Staph, Sul.

Oxaluria (excreation of urine containing calcium oxalate crystals: Berb v, Caust, Coca, Kali s, Lyco, Lycopus, Lysidin, Nat p, Nit ac, Nit mur ac, Ox ac, Plumb, Senna, Tereb, Zinc.

<u>PREVENTIVE MEDICINE</u>

- **Abdomen operation** – Rhus t 6x every 2 hours
- **Abortion** – Kali c 1M
- **Abortion** – Fight / anger – Acon
- **Abrasion due to walking** – Agnu cast
- **Appendicitis** – Psorinum 200 or CM, Cad iod, Bapt CM
- **Appendicitis –Trauma** – Arn
- **Air sickness-** Cocc
- **Alopecia areata** – Fl ac and Bac
- **Animal bites and boils** – Anthar
- **Arthritis** – Acet spicata, caulophyllum, Gaul
- **Bad effects of vaccination, small pox** – Maland
- **Bed wetting** – Apoc
- **Burns / scalds** – Canth
- **Cattaract** – Calc fl, Cineraria m
- **Cholera** – Camph
- **Chicken pox-** Ant t, Rhus t
- **Cold** – Amm c, Cistus can, Nux v
- **Collapse** – Carb v
- **Coryza** – Acon
- **Concussion, wisdom tooth** – Arn
- **Dental complication** – Hecla lava
- **Dentition** – Calc
- **Diptheria** – Diph
- **Dengu fever** – Eup perf
- **Dog bite** – Hydro phobinum
- **Epilepsy** – Ig, Amyl nit
- **Examination tension** – Lyc
- **Fractures** – Calc p
- **Formation of gall stones** – Chino
- **Gall stone** – Chol

- **Gangilon** – Ruta
- **Gangren** – Ars
- **Gonorrhoea** – Med
- **Gout** – Colchi
- **Grey hair** – Thyr, Acid p, Lyco, Phos, Pilocarpus.
- **Hair dyes** – Sulph
- **Haemorrhoides,varicose venis**- Ham
- **Hay fever** – Psor
- **Head injury** – Arn
- **Headeche** – Carb v, Cascara cord
- **Hernia** – Cocc
- **Hiccup** – Cajjuputam
- **Hormonal Balance**: Adren,Agnus, Insulin, Oophorinum, Orchitinum, Pitutarinum, Steroid hormone (parathyroid), Testosteron, Thyrodinum.
- **Hydrophobia** – Bell, Hyosc
- **Infection of the gland /eyes**- Staph
- **Influenza and cold** – Influ
- **Insect** – Apis
- **Jaundice** – Chin
- **Kdny stone** – Calc ren
- **Lckjaw**- Hyper
- **Lice** – Bac
- **Malaria** – Malar
- **Mania or phobia** – Alumina
- **Marasmus** – Iodi
- **Measles** – Puls, Morbillinum
- **Melancholia** – Kali p
- **Minor burns** – Utric u
- **Mosquito bites** – Led
- **Mumps** – Parotidinum
- **Typhoid** – Bapt

- **Shortens attack** – Morb
- **Syphilitic tissue** – Staph
- **Plague** – Ign
- **Whoophing cough** – Dros
- **Tonsillectomy** – Bar c
- **Snake Poison** – Euph
- **Styes recurring** – Hep
- **Pain ful labour** – Caul
- **Piles** – Tuber
- **Polio** – Lath
- **Post operative** – Stront c
- **Radiation** – Rad br
- **Radium burn** – Cad i
- **Rickets** – Thyr
- **Rubella (german measles)** – Puls 6
- **Sea sickness** – Tabacum
- **Small pox** – Variolinum
- **Stage firght** – Gels
- **Sun stroke** –Glon
- **Suppuration** – Pyrog and Sul ac
- **Stings** – Allium cepa
- **Tartar** – Calc ren
- **TB** – Ars iod
- **Tetanus** – Led and Hyper
- **Travel sickness** – Coca , Ign
- **Tobacco/ Coffe/ Alcohol/ opium and chloroform** – Aect ac
- **Tootheache** – Plantgo
- **Urine comes away drop by drop** – Lac d
- **Water in brain** – Sul 6, Calc p 6, Aur mur nat
- **Warts** – Fl ac, Nit ac
- **Whisky** – Puls

- **Whoophing cough** – Cupr ac, pertussoion
- **Worms** – Cina
- **Xray burns** – Cad i
- **Youth full looks** – Brewer's Yeast 1x, Ginkgo, Thiosinamnum.

<u>SURGERY & HOMEOPATHIC THERAPEUTICS</u>

Abscess: Hep, Merc s, Sul, Sul ac, Sil, Graph, Dulc, Ars a, Kali p, Fluo ac, Tub, Lach.

Acute Abdomen: Colocy, Mag p, Cheli, Beri v, Bell, Arn, Acon.

Appendicities: Ars, Bell, Carb veg, Cinchona, Gratiola, Kali bi, Lach, Puls, Phos.

Bell's Palsy: Bell, Cadmiun sul, Caust, Kali m, Pulmb, Picr ac, Rhus t, Stramonium, Tern.

Bile duct and Gall Blader: chinoth, Cheli, Lyco, Beri v, Merc, Nux v, Calc c, Phos, Crota h.

Bladder Atonic and Neurogenic: Caust, Gelsi, Ars a, Cicuta virosa,Plumb, Alumina.

Boils: Graph, Psori, Bell, Flour ac, Hep, Sili, Merc s, Ars.

Bones: Asafoetida, Calc c, Mez, Phyto, Ruta, Staph, Symphy, Calc p, Kali bi.

Brests: Con, Bryt c, Hydrast, Iod, Calc c, Calc fl, Lapis alb,

Burns: Aconit, Canth, Arn, Caust, Calendula, Ars.

Cataract: Phos, Arn, Lyco, Caust, Sil, Plumb,

Cervical Spondylosis: Spig, Ruta, Led, Arn, Acon, Gelsi, Theridion,

Colon: Chamomilla, Ipec, Colocy, Ars a, Nux v, Kali c, Cinchona.

Cornea: Aco, Euphra, Sabadi, Kali hyd, Calc c, Gelsi.

Cystitis: Canth, Lach, Chimphi, Campho, Cannabis in, Sarsaparilla, Pareira bra.

Duodenitis: Kali bi, Arg nit, Lyco, Hydrast, Phos, Nat mur, Tarent.

Dysuria: Coccus cac, Benz ac, Anthra, Calc c, Cannabis in, Ly co, Lithi c.

Epididymitis /Orchitis: Acon, Arn, Bell, Rhodo, Nit ac, Puls, Aur m.

Fistula: Thuj, Calc c, Merc s, Phos, Nit ac, Sil.

Glaucoma: Bell, Phos, Gelsi, Cedr, Sul, Acon, Phyto,

Gangrene: Secal cor, Carb veg, Brom, Ars a, Crot h, Eupho, Arn,

Gastricts: Bismuth, Kali c, Podo, Bry, Geranium maculatum, Carb veg, Ars a,

Goiter: Iod, Thyrodi, Bell, Calc c, Con, Lycopus, Nat m,

Haemorrhoids/Piles: Aloes, Mille, Hmamelis, Graph, Phos, Carb veg, Sul.

Heamiplegia: Alumina, Caust, Plumb m, Sil, Nux v, Physostg

Hernia: Canth, Alumina, Phos, Calc c, Lyco, Nux v,

Meningitis: Bell, Cicuta, Solium n, Gelsi, Gloni, Opium, Verat v.

Nasal Polyp: Calc c, Teucr mar, Kreosotum, Lemn m, Phos, Hamamelli.

Neuralgia: Stannum, Terbinth, Bell, Colocy, Phos, Agricus m,Nux v, Caust.

Otorrhoea: Ars a, Puls, Tellu, Psori, Kali bi, Lach, Mur ac, Merc s.

Peritonitis: Arn, Bell, Colocy, Lach, Lyco, Apis.

Prostate: Thuj, Con, Apis, Digi, Calc c, Bryt c, Staph, Chimphi.

Renal stones: Beri v, Sarasapa, Pareira br, Asparagus off, Calc c, Ocimum can, Canth.

Tootheache /teeth/ Odantalgia: Merc, Kreosotum, Puls, Staph, Mez, Lach, Calc c.

Tonsillitis: Lach, Baryt c, Merc s, Bell, Psori, Hep, Phos, Calc c.

Trauma wonds: Hyper, Arn, Calend, Ruta, Symphyt, Led, Staph, Rhus t, Phyto, Bufo.

A Genious Physician Leaves the Uric acid deposits in Blood and tissues: Colchicum

Removed Sciatica: Glinicum

Stiffness and Gout: Aconite

Morning Scikness: Meddorrhinum 1000

Cured Prolapsus / Fistula and Fissure: Nit ac

Bleeding cancer: Arsenic

Utren tumors: Aur mur nat

Acute Gout: Utrica urens

Ring worm: Baccillinum

Physical wrecks to health: Vanadium and Bellis per

Old people: Ferr p

Young: Acid flour

SURGERY & RECOVERY SUPPORT

Primary Remedies:

Arnica montana

This remedy relieves pain, bruising and swelling associated with trauma, surgery or overexertion.

Bellis perennis

This remedy is useful when bruising and trauma occur to deep internal tissues after surgery involving the abdomen, breasts, or trunk-especially if a feeling of stiffness or coldness has developed in the area.

Hypericum perforatum

This remedy relieves pain that seems to follow the nerve's path.

Ledum palustre

Ledum palustre relieves bruising around wounds from pointed objects.

Phosphorus

This remedy may be helpful if a person has trouble recovering from the effects of anesthesia. Symptoms can include disorientation, stupor, weakness, nausea and vomiting. The person may be thirsty but often vomits after drinking.

Staphysagria

This remedy relieves itching or pain in surgical or clean cut wounds, and warts.

Other Remedies:

Aconitum apellus

This remedy is indicated when people anticipating surgery are extremely agitated or panicked, especially if they fear that they will die. Easy startling, a sensitivity to light and noise, dry mouth, and thirst are other indications for *Aconitum*.

Causticum

This remedy relieves painful scars from burns, with thin and fragile skin, especially in elderly patients.

Cinchona officinalis

This homeopathic remedy relieves weakness due to loss of fluids (diarrhea, bleeding and sweating), with gas in the abdomen.

Coffea cruda

This relieves sleeplessness with worries, overactive thoughts, and hypersensitivity to pain.

Ferrum phosphoricum

This remedy is helpful for early stages of any inflammation and may reduce the chance of soreness and infection after surgery.

Gelsemium

This remedy can be helpful to a person who feels nervous fear before an operation, with trembling, lethargy, and often diarrhea or headache.

Graphites

This remedy reduces thick scars.

Hamamelis

This remedy can help with passive bleeding if a person's veins are weak, and may also relieve discomfort after surgery on varicose veins and hemorrhoids.

Rhus toxicodendron

This remedy is helpful for relief of stiffness, soreness, and restlessness after any surgery. It is often recommended after operations on tonsils and adenoids, appendectomy, and dental surgery.

Ruta graveolens

This remedy is often useful after surgeries involving tendons, connective tissue, cartilage, joints, and coverings of the bones. It can ease discomfort and promote recovery after surgery on knees, wrists, shoulders, elbows, ankles, hips, etc. It may also be soothing if deep stiffness is felt in joints and muscles after surgery.

Thuja occidentalis

This remedy relieves skin lesions that tend to protrude (warts or thick scars).

Silicea

This relieves symptoms of general fatigue with chilliness, lack of energy and irritability.

Dilation and curettage: **Belladonna 30**, every 6 hours

–Hysterectomy: **Causticum 30**, three times a day (some homeopaths recommend **Staphysagria 6 or 30**, three times a day)

–Caesarean section or episiotomy: **Staphysagria 30** or **Bellis perennis 30**, three times a day

–Abortion or miscarriage: **Ignatia 30**, every four hours

–Plastic surgery on the breast: **Bellis perennis 6 or 30**, three times a day

–Amputation of the breast or a lump: **Hamamelis 30**, every 4 hours

Circumcision: **Staphysagria 30** and **Arnica 30**, every four hours for a day.

Prostate surgery: **Staphysagria 30**, three times a day

Abdominal surgery: **Staphysagria 30** or **Bellis perennis 30**, three times a day

Appendectomy: **Rhus tox 30**, three times a day

Gastrectomy: **Raphanus 30**, three times a day

Gall bladder surgery: **Lycopodium 30**, three times a day

Eye surgery: **Ledum 30**, every four hours

Tonsillectomy and adenoidectomy: **Rhus tox 30**, every four hours

Orthopedic surgery

–involving cartilage or periosteum: **Ruta 30**, every four hours

–involving the spine: **Hypericum 30**, every four hours

–Surgery for bullet wounds and/or stab wounds: **Staphysagria 30**, four times a day

Plastic surgery: **Arnica 30** (internally) and **Calendula**, (externally) four times a day

Amputation: **Hypericum 30**, every four hours

Hemorrhoids: **Staphysagria 30** or **Aesculus 30**, every four hours for two or three days* Varicose veins: **Ledum 30**, three times a day

Dental surgery: **Hypericum 30** and **Ruta 30**, alternating every two to four hours

<u>RARE OBSERVATIONS</u>

Death fear: Ars alb, Digit, Gelsi, Lac can

No fear of death: Lac d

Eats every few hours: cina, iodium, sulph

Eats well but weight loss: Abrot, iod, Nat m, Saniquila

Head nodding : Sepia

Frequent winking: Staph

Tobbaco caving : Daphne

Snake tongue: Lachesis

Ittching without irrupations: Dolichos

Fidgety feet: Zin

Constant Swallowing: Sabadilla

Near sweating: Nux m

Regurgitating: Lyco

Mountain loving: Syphi

Sea loving: Bromium

Salt craving: Nat mur

Sweet craving: Arg nit

Darkness fearing: Strom

Midnight hungry: Psorinum

Thrstless: Puls

Head sweats- Body is dry: sil

Body sewats Head is dry: Rhus t

Flatulence: Carb veg, China, Lyco

Burning sensation: Ars alb, Phos, Sulph

Pain: Aconite, Chamomi, Coffea

Delirium: Bell, Hyscya, Stram

Effects of gref: Ig, Nat m, Acid phos

Rheumatism: Caust, Rhu t, Sulph

Taste: Acid m (everthing sweet), Ars alb (taste salty & water teste bitter), Bell & Sep (salt), Bovista & Sul (blood), Hydra (Piper), Iod (soap), Lyco (sour), Myristic seb (coppery), Puls (nothing taste), Carb v(greasy),

Lock Jaw: Campho, Hyper, Ledum, Mag p, Nux v, Pssi f, Strychinium p, Vetram v.

Thalassemia: Antipyrinum, Ars alb, Butryricum acid 1x,Calc ars, Ferr m, Lach, Phos, Pic ac, Pluymb m, Thiosinaminum, Thyrodi.

HOMEOPATHIC NOSODES INCLUDE:

Anthracinum (Anthr.): Anthracinum works for carbuncles that are blue and burning.

Bacillinum(Bac.): **Tuberculosis** Bacillinum is used for weak lungs of elderly people and for children with chronic catarrhal conditions and attacks of suffocation at night with difficult cough and chronic catarrhal conditions

Borrelia   burgdorferi: (Lyme   nosode) This nosode is used for homeopathic immunization for Lyme disease.

Carcinosin (Carc.): Breast Cancer Tissue

Diphtherinum (Diph.) Nosode: This nosode is used for homeopathic immunization for diphtheria.

Folliculinum (Foll.): This nosode is made from estrogen. It can be an important remedy for women who have estrogen poisoning as a result of using birth control pills. Folliculinum is also used in an acute type of treatment in women to regain their fertility and ovulation cycle again after a period of it being suppressed by the usage the birth control pills.

Haemophilus: Hib Influenza, Type B This nosode is used for homeoprophylaxis and treatment of Hib Influenza Type B.

Histaminum hydrocholoricum: The nosode is made from histaminum hydrochloricum, a kind of histamine used as a homeopathic remedy used for allergies.

Influenzinum (Influ.): This nosode is used for homeopathic immunization for influenza (flu.)

Lathyrus Sativus: Polio This is the homeopathic remedy used to prevent **polio.**

Lyssin (Hydrophobinum): Rabies This nosode is used for homeopathic immunization for rabies.

Medorrhinum (Medh.): Gonnorhea This nosode is made from gonorrhea. It is a very important remedy for hormonal problems.

Meningococcinum: **Meningitis** **bacteria.** This nosode is used for homeopathic immunization for meningitis. **Morbillinum (Morbill.): Measles (rubeola) virus.** This nosode is used for homeopathic immunization for measles.

Oscillococcinum (Oscillo.): Duck heart and liver This nosode is used for homeopathic immunization for influenza (flu.) Oscillococcinum is a nosode made from duck heart and liver.

Parotidinum (Parot.): Mumps virus. This nosode is used for homeopathic immunization for mumps.

Pertussin (Pert.): Pertussis (whooping cough) This nosode is used for homeopathic immunization for pertussis (whooping cough)

Pneumococcinum: **Puenmococcoal** **bacteria.** This nosode is used for homeopathic immunization for pneumococcal disease.

Psorinum (Psor.): Scabies discharge. This nosode is made from a scabies discharge and is used in homeopathic prescribing.

Rubella: German measles (rubella). This nosode is used for homeopathic immunization of German measles.

Scarlatinum (Scarlatininum) This is a homeopathic nosode prepared from Scarlatina or Scarlet Fever.

Staphyloconum (Staphycoc.): Staphylococcus bacteria This nosode is made from staphylococcus, a group of bacteria that can cause a multitude of diseases as a result of infection of various tissues of the body.

Streptococcinum (Streptoc.): Streptococcus bacteria This nosode is made from streptococcus and is used when there is strep in the person's history and it has been suppressed with antibiotics.

Syphilinum (Syphil.): Syphilis The nosode is made from syphilis. It is used for chronic conditions such as asthma, constipation, painful menstruation, inflammation of the iris and neuralgia. Symptoms appear gradually and resolve slowly.

Tetanus Toxin: Tetanus This nosode is used for homeopathic immunization of tetanus.

Tuberculinum (Tub.): Tuberculosis The nosode is made from the sputum of a tubercular person.

Varicella Zoster: Chicken Pox This nosode is used for homeopathic immunization of chicken pox.

Variolinum: Small Pox This nosode is used for homeopathic immunization of small pox.

Most of the nosodes listed below are not listed in the pharmacopoeia, hence standardization is suspect.

- **Agaricus Muscaris** – entire fresh fungus found in dry pinewoods.
- **Ambra Grisea** – morbid secretion from the liver of Spermaceti Whale (Physeter Macrocephalus).
- **Anti-Colibacillary-** purified form of stock serum anti-colibacillary of caprine origin, made from goats immunized with E.coli.
- **Boletus Laricis-** prepared from dried fungus Purging Agaric / Larch Boletus.
- **Botulinum-** Clostridium Botulinum toxin made from putrefied pork.

- **Brucella Melintensis-** a filtrate of a 21 days old culture of the microbe of undulating fever.
- **Calculus bilialis**
- **Calculus renalis-** prepared from renal calculus.
- **Cholesterinum** – prepared from gall stone.
- **Colibacillinum**
- **D.T.-T.A.B.-** mixed vaccine of antidiphtheric, antitetanic and antitypho – paratyphoid.
- **Eberthinum-** prepared from culture of mixture of many stocks of Salmonella typhi.
- **Enterococcinum-** stocks of Streptococcus faecalis.
- **Flavus-** prepared from Neisseria pharangis.
- **Gonotoxinum-** prepared from anti Gonococcic vaccine.
- **Hippomanes-** prepared from a sticky mucoid substance of urinous odour found in the amniotic fluid of the mare. It is also found attached to the membrane of the foetal organ of the mare in last month of pregnancy.
- **Hippozaenium-** lysate from the glander of horse.
- **Homarus**
- **Hydrophobinum** (Lyssin)- lysate of saliva taken from a rabid dog.
- Leprominum
- Leprum
- Leptospira- lysate of Leptospira ictero-haemorrhagie
- Leusinum (Syphilinum)- prepared from serosity of Trepanoma pallidum of syphilitic chancres.
- Malandrinum- lysate from exudates of the horse malandra: discharge of eczema in the fold of the knee of horse.
- Malaria Officinalis- prepared from mire taken during dryness of a malarial marsh.
- Medorrhinum- purulent urethral secretion taken during the period of discharge infected with Neisseria Gonorrhoeae.
- Melitagrinum- nosode of Eczema capitis
- Meningococcinum- prepared from stocks of Neisseria Meningitidis.
- Monilia Albicans- lysate of culture of Monilia albicans

- Morbillinum- from exudate of mouth and pharynx of measles affected patients
- Mucor Mucedo- lysate obtained by isolating and transplanting the mushroom Mucor Mucedo from the medium of culture.
- Mucotoxin
- Nectrianinum- nosode of Cancer of trees.
- Oscillococcinum- autolysate filtered from liver and heart of a duck.
- Osteo Arthritis Nosode (O.A.N.)- synovial fluid of articulations especially knee and hip of osteoarthritic patients.
- Ourlianum- lysate from the saliva of a patient suffering from mumps.
- Paratyphoidinum- prepared from cultures from mixture of different stocks of Paratyphoidinum bacilli.
- Pertussinum- lysate from expectoration of patient suffering from whooping cough.
- Pneumococcinum- Diplococcus pneumoniae found in saliva
- Pneumotoxin- prepared from Diplococcus lanceolatus.
- Psorinum- lysated stock obtained from serosity of furrows of itch of an unterated patient.
- Pulmo anaphylacticus
- Putrescinum
- Pyrarara- lard of Pyrarara, a fish of the Amazon river.
- Pyrogenum- prepared originally from decomposition of meat of beef.
- Rheumatoid Arthritis Nosode (R.A.N)- prepared from synovial fluid of knee afflicted with rheumatoid arthritis
- Sanguisuga- prepared from leech.
- Scarlatinum- lysate from the scabs of a patient suffering from scarlatina.
- Secale Cornutum- prepared from the fungus Claviceps purpura.

- Serum of Yersin- from the anti-pest serum obtained from animals that have been immunized by means of live or killed cultures of Yersinia pestis.
- Septicaeminum – prepared from septic abscess.
- Sinusitisinum
- Staphylococcinum- lysate of culture of many stocks of Staphylococcus pyogenes aureus.
- Staphylotoxinum- antitoxins of staphylococcus.
- Streptococcinum- lysate obtained from stock of streptococcus.
- Streptoenterococcinum- lysate of culture of strepto-enterococcus.
- Tetanotoxinum – dilution of tetanic toxin.
- Toxoplasma Gondii – lysate of Toxoplasma Gondii.
- Ustilago Maydis- prepared from a fungus growing on the Indian corn.
- Usnea Barbata – prepared from lichen infecting soft maple.
- Vaccin attenu bili
- Vaccinotoxinum- prepared from anti-variolic vaccine.
- Vaccinonum- prepared from the lymph of cowpox.
- Variolinum- lysate obtained from the serosity of smallpox pustule.
- Verriculum- prepared from warts.
- Yersin (Pestinum)- nosode of plague.

Carcinosins Nosodes in Homeopathy:

- Epitheliomine – extract of epithelioma.
- Schirrinum- carcinoma schirrus (stomach).
- Onkolysine- from a stock of Onkomyxa Neojormans.
- Carcinosin-hepatica-metastat
- Carcinosin laryngis
- Carcinosin adenopapillary
- Carcinosin adeno-stom- from adenocarcinoma of stomach.
- Carcinosin adeno-vesica- papillary adenocarcinoma of bladder.
- Carcinosin pulmonale- pulmonary cancer.

- Carcinosin Schirr-mammae- schhirus of mammae.

Tuberculinums are Nosodes In Homeopathy:

- Tuberculinum avis- prepared from Mycobacterium tuberculosis aviaire.
- Tuberculinum bovinum- prepared from the pus of tuberculosis abscess.
- Tuberculinum Koch- culture of Mycobacterium tuberculosis.
- Tuberculinum Marmoreck- obtained from horses vaccinated by the filtrates of young cultures of Tuberculosis bacilli.
- Tuberculinum laricus
- Tuberculinum residuum Koch
- Bacillinum Burnett- from the sputum of tuberculosis patients containing the bacteria.
- Bacillinum testium- prepared from the testicle of tuberculosis patient.
- Diluted B.C.G.- from vaccine B.C.G.

Other Nosodes

- Actinomyces
- Adenoidum
- Arteriosclerosis
- Bacillus pyocyanaeus
- Bilharzia
- Brucella melitensis
- Cysticercosis
- Egg vaccine
- Epihysterinum
- Framboesinum
- Haffkine
- Osseinum
- Ringworm

<u>EMERGENCY FOR HOMEOPATHY</u>
<u>First AID:</u>

- **Anaphylaxis:** Acon; Apis.
- **Bites and stings:** Apis; Arn; Canth; Led.
- **Blisters:** Canth; Rhus-t.
- **Bruises:** Arn; Led.
- **Burns and scalds:** Canth; Urt-u.
- **Cuts, scrapes and puncture wounds:** Arn; Calend; Hyper; Led.
- **Dental Work:** Arn; Hyper; Ruta.
- **Electroshock:** Phos.
- **Eye injuries:** Arn; Led; Euphr; Symph.
- **Food poisoning:** Ars; Nux-v.
- **Fractures:** Arn; Symph.
- **Heat stroke or exhaustion:** Bell; Glon.
- **Hyperventilation:** Acon.
- **Motion sickness:** Cocc; Tabac.
- **Nosebleeds:** Arn; Phos.
- **Overindulgence and hangover:** Nux-v
- **Panic and Shock:** Acon.
- **Poison Ivy:** Rhus-t.
- **Splinters and thorns:** Sil.
- **Sprains and strains:** Arn; Hyper; Led; Rhus-t; Ruta.

Bites

- When there is swelling and bruising.- Arnica
- In sect Stings.- Apis mel
- Horse-fly bites.- Hypericum
- Purple discoloration around the bite.- Lachesis
- Pain from puncture wounds from small sharp objects.- Ledum
- Mosquito bites –Staphasagria
- Swollen bites that itch and sting-Utrica uren

Bleeding

Crot. H. – haemorrhagic diathesis, hemorrhage from every orifice, from nose, mouth, ears, anus, vagina, uterus, bowels, lungs, and from all mucus membranes. Intraocular hemorrhage; all discharges are bloody, even sweat and saliva are bloody.Purpura haemorrhagica, comes on suddenly, from all orifices, skin, nails and gums. Blood is dark, fluid and non coaguable; hemorrhage occurring in typical zymotic disease and Ammonium Carb, Arnica Montana, China, Kali Mur, Veratrum album, Belladonna ,Lachesis, Hamamelis, Carbo veg, Ferrum, Phosphorous, Sulphuric acid etc…

Boils

- With redness, heat and throbbing – Belladonna
- Sensitive boils which weep easily – Hepar sulph
- Boils slow to develop and heal – Silicea

Broken Bones

- Arnica: Broken bones typically come with a degree of blunt trauma to soft tissues – which in turn leads to swelling, pain and discoloration.
- Eupatorium perfoliatum: This homeopathic remedy is well-known for its use in flu and fever when the patient feels pains in the bones ("as if broken") and can be useful to relieve the deep or aching pain of actual broken bones.
- Hypericum: This homeopathic remedy is very useful for crushing injuries to body areas that are well-supplied with nerves like fingers and toes.
- Ruta graveolens: This homeopathic remedy is known for its effect on bone-bruises and on injuries to the periosteum (the covering of the bones); both of these types of trauma are involved when a fracture of a bone occurs.
- Symphytum officinale: this homeopathic remedy is often a great help in accelerating callous formation (bone repair) after a break and it can also help relieve the pain of a break.

Chickenpox

Acon., ant-c., ant-t., ars., asaf., bell., canth., carb-v., caust., coff., con., cycl., hyos., ip., led., merc., nat-c., nat-m., puls., rhus-t., sep., sil., sulph., thuj.

Cuts, Scrapes & Open Wounds

Bellis perennis, Arnica, Calendula, Hypericum, Ledum, & Ruta medicines and creams

Choking: Bryt c, Cactus, Laches, Mephitis, Spigelia

Diarrhea

Podophyllum, Colocynthis, Nux Vomica, Arsenicum Album, Ipecacuanha.

Electrocution and Shocks

- Electroshock, electricity agg - arn., hell., morph., nux-v., Phos. ailments from - hell., morph., phos.
- Burns - canth.
- Convulsions - complete unconsciousness, with - Hell.consciousness, with - Nux-v.
- Dream-like state, with - Morph.
- Lightning strikes - morph, Nux -v., op. phos.
- Blindness from lighting - phos.
- Simple shocks - Arn.
- Susceptibility, great, to electric shocks - Phos.
- Unconsciousness, complete - Hell.

Emergency Life saving drug: Camphora, Carbo Vegetabilis, Strontium carbonicum.

Fevers

1. <u>Dengue:</u> Aconitum napellus – high fever (redness of face), severe headache, cold sweat, thirst for water. Echnacea angustofolia 1x Tablets: anti-inflammatory, anti-viral activity. And Bryonia alba, Eupatorium perfoliatum, Rhus Toxicodendron.

2. <u>Chikungunya:</u> Eupatorium perfolatum –Wonderful homeopathic remedy for all kind of joint and muscles pain developed with or after febrile disease. Bone pains, general to severe and Rhus toxicodendron, China, Pyroginum, Arnica, Arsenic album.

3. <u>Swine Flu:</u> Gelsemium. [Gels], Baptisia. Eupatorium perfoliatum., Sabadilla. [Sabad], Arsenicum. [Ars], Arsenicum iodide. Dulcamara. [Dulc], Bryonia, Phosphorus, Rhus toxicodendron. [Rhus-t], Allium cepa. [All-c], Sticta. [Stict], Ipecac, Veratrum albu.

4. <u>Typhoid:</u> Baptisia, Bryonia, Rhus toxicodendron, Arnica, Arsenicum, cinchona, Carbo vegetabilis, Lachesis, Kali phosphoricum, Gelsemium, Phosphoric acid.

5. <u>Malaria:</u> Arnica, Arsenicum,Belldona, Carbo vegetabilis, Eupatorium perfoliatum, China, Ipecac, Natrum Mur.

Food Poisoning:

- Arsenicum: Bad effects of spoiled fish, meat and bad water. Burning pain in abdomen, person feels chilly, restless, anxious, thirsty for sips of water. Vomiting and diarrohea at the same time. Better for warmth and warm drinks, worse from cold drinks and sight or smell of food.

- Lycopodium: Bad effects of shellfish especially oysters.

- Pulsatilla: Stomach disorders from eating cakes, rich foods, ice-cream, spoiled meats and rotten fish.

- Nux Vomica: Bad effects of overindulgence in food and wine, fatty foods, spicy foods and alcohol. Symptoms of cramps, hangovers, wind, pressure, and vomiting which does not relieve.

- Urtica Urens: Ailments from eating shellfish with allergic skin reaction.

- China: This it an excellent remedy to help promote recovery after fluid loss which has arisen because of symptoms such as persistent sweating, vomiting, diarrohea causing exhaustion and dehydration.

- Rehydration is essential to replace the enormous amounts of fluids lost during food poisoning.

Homeopathic First-aid Remedies for Heart Attack

- Aconitum napellus: Use when the patient has difficulty breathing, is anxious, but feels better sitting up.

- Cactus grandiflorus: When the attack strikes between approximately noon and midnight, feels as if something is "squeezing" the heart or the pain is severe enough to make the patient cry, shout or whimper.

- Digitalis: This remedy is indicated when symptoms include blue skin, numbness and weakness of the left arm, a slow pulse and great fear.

Homeopathic Knief: Myristica seb, Heper sul, Sili.

Jaws: Hekla Lava.

Nosebleed: Agar., Amyl, Ant. c., Ham., Meli.

Sprains

- Sprain coupled with bruising – Arnica

- Sprain painful for movement – Bryonia

- Pain improved by gentle movement – Rhus tox

- Sprain with bone injury - Ruta grav

Sun Stroke

- Nowadays gradually rising of temperature lends a common condition known as sun stroke or heat stroke. In which extreme high temperature up to 47°C (106°F) with scanty sweating and profuse fluid loss due to diarrhea & vomiting is common. In such situation use of modern allopathic drugs like acetaminophen, NSAIDS may become harmful to decrease temperature because of imbalance in hypothalamus that medicines may lead to hepatic or renal toxicity.

- **Homeopathy medicines:** Aconite N, Belladonna, Glonoine, Natrum Carb, Veratrum Viride.

Traumatic: Acon., Arn., Bell., Hyper., Nat. s., Sil.

COMMUNICABULE DISEASES

HIV & AIDS: Ars I, Ars a, Baccili, Calc io, Crtolus h, Kali c, Silicia, Sulphur, Tuber, Syphilinum, Phos, Vanadi, Zin m.Nux vom, Psorinum, Merc sol, Thuja, Nitric acid, Medo, Acon, Carbo veg, Rhustox

Malaria Fever: Cina 30, Ipecac 30, Ars 30

Simple Continued Fever: Sulp 200+ Pyrogi200

Typhoid: Pyrogi 200, Tyrodi 200

Influezia: Bryonia 30, Eup perf 30, Gelsi 30

Scarlatia: Bryonia 30,Gelsi 30, Bell 30

Yellow Fever: Ars 30, Lachsi 30, Crotalus 30

Black wter fever: Nat m, Cimex 30, Calc ars 30

Measels: Bry 30, Melend 30, Ars 30

Small pox: Ant t 30, Varolinum 30, Hepr sul 30

Chiken pox: Sili 6x, Kali p 6x, Ferr p 6x

Pneumonia: Bry 30, sul 30, Phos 30

Pelurasy: Heper sul 200, Phos 200

Diptheria: Callus 30, Phytolacca 30, Bell 30

Mumps: Bell 200, Merc s 200

Plumonary TB: Cina 30, Ipec 30, Ars 30

Scrofula: Bart c 30, Ars iod 30, Conium m 30

Meningits: Cicuta ver 30, Apis 30, Bry 30

Plage: Pyroginum 30, Hydrocyanic ac 30, Pestunium 30

Whoophing cough: Bell 200, Drosera 200, Baccili 200

Dysentary: Merc c 30, Podophi 30, Ars 30

Cholera: Camphor 30, Cup m 30, Verat alb 30

Hydrophobia: Lyssinum 200,Stramonium 200, Hyos nig 200

Leprosy: Hydro c 30, Ars iod 30, Graph 30

Tetnus: Ledum 30, Hyperi 30, Cicuta 30

<u>VACCATION FOR CHILDHOOD DISEASES</u>

Chicken Pox Prevention: Rhus toxicodendron & Varicella Zoster (Prevention), Anti t, Anti c, Apis, Bell, Bry, Merc s, Mezer, Puls, Sul, Utri u.

Diphtheria: Diphtherium (Prevention), Apis, Ars, Bapti,Brom ,Calc f, Calc p, Calc ac, Ferr p, Kali bich, Kali m, Kali p, Kali per, Lac c, Lach, Lyco, Merc, Muratic ac, Nat m ,Nat p, Nat s, Nitr ac, Phyto, Rhus t.

Hepatitis B: Hepatitis B

Influenza: Influenzinum, Oscillococcinum, Acon, Anti t, Ars a, Bapt, Bray, Chemo, Dulc, Eup perf, Euphr, Ferr p, Gelsi, Ipec, Nux v, Puls, Verat alb.

Measles: Morbillinum,Puls, Euphr, Acon, Apis, sul, Bell, Bry, Kali bi.

Meningitis
Symptoms Include:
- Convulsions
- Floppy and unresponsive, or stiff with jerky movements
- Irritable and not wanting to be held
- Loss of appetite
- Pale and blotchy skin
- Staring expression
- Swelling in the soft part of their head (fontanelle).
- Unusual crying
- Very sleepy with a reluctance to wake up
- Vomiting and refusing feeds

Homeopathy Remedies: Acon, Apis, Bell, Bapt, Bray, Camphor, Cineria m, Cicuta, Gelsi, Cup m, Hellebo n, Podo, Sul, Utri u, Verat v, Zin m.

Mumps : Parotidinum, Acon, Bell, Coni, Lach, Merc s, Phyto, Jaborandi, Puls, Rhus t.

Pertussis, Whooping Cough: Pertussin,Acon, Anti t, Arn, Cina, Cup m, Corralium r, Cacus c, Drosera, Bell, Heper s, Ipec, Kali bi, Ledum, Mag p, Sul.

Pneumococcal Disease:

Symptoms of bacterial pneumonia **develop abruptly** and may include:

- **Breathing may become labored and heavy** (in advanced cases)
- **Chest pain**
- **Chills**
- Coughing up **sputum containing pus or blood** in advanced cases, indication of serious infection)
- **Fever**
- Person may become confused (in advanced cases)
- **Rapid breathing and heart beat**
- **Severe abdominal pain** may accompany pneumonia occurring in the lower lobes of the lung.
- **Shaking**
- **Shortness of breath**

Homeopathy remedies: Acon, Anti t, Cheli, Ferr p, Iodium, Bry, Kali m, Lyco, Merc s, Phos, Sang, Sul, Verat v.

Polio: Gelsi, Lathurus sativa.

Rotavirus: Rotavirus Nosode

Tetanus: Ledum, Ars, Acon, Angustu vera, Camphor, Cup met, Cicuta, Hydrocy ac, Hyper, Lach Nux v, Passi, Sil, Stramo, Strichi, Vtrum alb.

Rubella: Acon, Bell, Puls, Rubella

CHILDEREN DISEASES

Adenoides: Thuja, Varietal carb and Azhi iodide

Amoebiasis: podophylum, azhse, sina, abrotanum

Asthma- bronchitis: Sambucus,

Brings a boil to a head. Colds, sore throat or hoarseness with a sensation of a splinter in the throat: Hepar Sulphuris Calcareum 30C.

Barking cough sounds: Spong 30

Bruising. Muscular soreness – Arn 30

Continuous crying of the infant: Chamomilla 30.

Colic and teething pain: Chemmomi 30

Colds in children prone to otitis and bronchitis: Ferr p 30

Cuts & burning: Calend 30

Dental caris: Fluric acid, sepia

Fevers and inflammations: Acon 30

Hives and swelling; insect bites- Apis30

High fever of sudden onset with hot, red, flushed face red and sweating: Bell 30

Hyper Activity: Agricus mus, Agr nit, Ars a,Brayt c, Kali brom, Mag c, Tarent, Zinc m.

Influenza or cold: Bell 30, Acon 30, Bry 30, Nux v 30.

Infection: Heper s

Mouth full of saliva & Vomting: Ipec 30

Tonsillitis: Bell, Lyco and Bryt c

Polypus in the nose: Calcarea c, Sanguinaria, Canadensis, Hydrasti.

<u>ILL EFFECTS</u>

Breathlessness/insomnia: Coca

Chloroform: Chamomilla

Colic: Colocynth

Cold weather / hair cut: Bell

Cold winds / Mastrubation: Bellis p

Deafness: Cheiranthus

Driking tea: China off

Eating eegs: Chininum ars

Eye sight /masturbation: Cina

Effects of ice creams/Alchol/Watery fruts/ inhealing anthrax : Ars alb

Gout: Abrot

Head injury: Helleborus

Inhealing Carbon monaxied gas: Aceticum ac

Inhealing charcoal fumes: Amm c

Inhealing foul odor: Anthracinum

X ray: Acid f, Radium bro, Cadmium iod, Silicia

Loss of semen or blood: Acid p

Loss of sleep or over work: Cocculus ind

Sexual desire: Conium

Swimming/ river bathing: Anti c

Typhoid fever: Bry alb

Working in water: Calc c

Shock: Camphora

Drinking too cold: Carb v, Kalli c

Vaccination: Malandrium, Sili. Thuja

Very cold bath: Dulcmara

Tooth extertion: Gun powder

Mental troubles: Nat sul

Salt: Phos

Atom bomb: Phos,Stromonium c

Poisning: Pyroginum

Bad food/ bad water: Sil

Over lifting: Rhus t, Formica r, Millifolium

Utrine diseas: Thalapsi

Eczima: Thuja

Hair dye: Tuberc

Spermatorrhea: Tribulus

PLASTIC SURGERY

Arms very lean: Gaph

Arms very red : Puls, Sulph

Back very big : Calc c, Bar c, Nux

Back very thin: Lach, Tabac

Belly very big: Puls, Nux, Calc c, Nat m.

Body circumference very big: Sulph, Nat m, Nat c.

Breast Disappeared in 18 years young womens: Iodium 200

Breast Disappeared in 49 years young womens: Staph sagria 200 or Iodium 200

Breasts disappeared (Skeletal thinness of the neck): Mercurius cyanatum

Deformed breasts after feeding or after delivery: Pulsatilla, Brynonia, Belladonna, Mercurius vivus.

Breast very small: Con, Nit ac, Ars, Sulph, Iod, Calc c, Ign, Puls, Carb v, Graph, Staph.

Breast not at developed in a girl of 24 years: Staph

Breast not sufficiently firm In a women of at 46 years: Graph, Iod

Breast very small with goitor: Calc c, Iod

-very voluminous: Calc c, Sulph, Nux, Nat m.

- Bell, Bry, Phos, Hep

Buttocks, hips, pelvis, very big: Bar c, Calc c, Anti c. Merc cy.

Buttocks, hips, pelvis, very thin: Sil, Lyc, Sulph, Graph.

Buttocks very big: Nux.

Cheeks very fat: Calc c, Sulph, Puls.

Checks very lean: Chin, Ph ac, Ars, Terbe.

Cheeks very red: Nux, Sulph, Calc c.

Cheeks hanging in old men: Sulph, Lyc, Sili, Bell, Nux, Ign, Rhus.

Eyes surrounded with blue aura: Staphysagria, China, Phosphoric acid.

Neck very short and very big, Enormous double chin: Nux. Vom

Obesity of belly: Nux-Vom. 200

Very great development of cheeks, breasts and the stature, Limbs very thin: Nux vomica

Breasts, tops of the shoulders, calves, figures, ephelides: Graphites 600

LIFESTYLE DISORDERS IN HOMEOPATHY

Addiction: Stramonium, Opium, Avena Sativa, Nux v, Qurecus g, Morphinum, Coffea, Sul ac, Hyosc.

Reduce alcohol cravings in others: Syphilinum, Sulphur

Assist with weaning off morphine or heroin: Bell, Avaina sativa.

Antitox (nicotine habit): Tabacum,Plantago

Antidots: Acet ac, Acid fl(radiation), Agricus muc(Alcohol), Alumen(lead poisoning), Ars alb(Pencilin & carbolic ac), Carb veg(fumens of gases), Chamomi(excessive coffe drinking), Graph(Skin troubles & arsnic poisoning), Insulin(Insulin), Ipec(quinine & opium poisoning), Ledum(poisons of animal insects), Nit ac (anti biotics), Nux v(Stimulates wine,whisky,tea,coffe), Phos & Amm c (chloropharm/anesthetic drugs), Thuja(vaccination), Tuber(hair dyes)

Alchoholism: Acid s, Angelia, China o, Phos, Quercus, Sepia, Kali bich,Sil, Sterculia a, Strychninum, Sul, Syphili 1M.

Ill effects of Alchoholism: Ars alb, Calc ars, Carb sul, Cardus, Chimphilla, Gclsi, Kalium bich, Nux v, Puls, Petrol, Quercus, Ranunculu b, Secle cor, Sili, Strophanthus.

Alzheimer's disease: Genkgo, Gensing, Aswagandha

Anxiety: Acon, Anac, Arg nit, Ars al, Borax, Bry al, Calc c, Carb veg, Caust, Gelsi, Ign, Laches, Lyco,Mag m, Nat m, Phos, Puls, Sepi, Sul.

Arteriosclerosis: Adrena, Cactus, Calc c, Cratagus oxy, Sumbulus, Thiosi, Thyrodi.

Blood Pressure: Bell, Gloni, Nux v, Nat m, Aurum m, Bryt c, Leches, Allu sati, Amyl nit, Rawulfolia, Adren

Cancer (mostly skin and lung): Calc-f, Lap-a,Sil, Hekla, Con, Condurango, Bryt c, Bryt iod, Phytol, Pumb iod, Ars, Bromine (mammary), Iodine (uters/hammorides), Radium brom, Carb ac, Carb an, Cedron.

Constipation: Bry, Nux, Nat m, Graph, Lyco, Sepia, Calc c, Caust, Sil, Sul, Chelido, Cardus.

Diabetes: Ars brom,Cephenadra indi, Syzigum, Glyserinum, Ozone, Uranium nit, Insulin, Curare, Acid p, Lac ac,

Diabetes Nuropathy: Con, Plumb, Calendula

Dust Allergy: Pothus, Ars al, Anti t, Euphra, Nat m, Sabadilla, Allium cepa, Wyethia.

Diabetes in fungal infection: Helonius, Kreostom

Hypothyroidism Calc phos., Calc c., Lapis alb., iodium., Thyroidinum, Spong., Lycopus, Calc-iod.

Insomnia (Sleeplessness): Gensing, Aswagandha, Arg nit, Coffie, Pisidia, Kali p.

Obesity: Calc c, Lyco, Amm mur, Amm c, Nat m, Anti c, Phytolacca, Graph, Nux v, Fucus.

Piles: Anacadi, Assculs hip, Hammamellis,Nux v, Sulp, Bry, Lyco, Carb v, Collinsonia, Ratanhia, Milli,paonea.

Stress: Aconite, Calcaria Carb, Lycopodium, Nux vom.

Renal failure: Apis, Ars, Aur Mur, Bell, Cantha, Convallaria.Cupr ars, Aur m, Cupr m, Opium, Terbenth, Phos.

<u>DIET & DISEASES</u>

<u>Diabetes mellitus:</u>

DO NOT:

- Skip meals.
- Eat heavy and fatty meals.
- Eat saturated fats such as butter, coconut oil and palm oil.
- Eat salty food.
- Choose foods that are high in sugar, such as cake, pie, doughnuts, sweetened cereal, honey, jam, jelly, ice cream, or candy.
- Choose sugar-sweetened beverages like sodas and fruit juices.
- Add sugar to your foods.

Do:

- Fatty Fish
- Leafy green
- Cinnamon
- Eggs
- Turmeric
- Greek yogurt
- Almonds: 2.6 grams
- Brazil nuts: 1.4 grams
- Cashews: 7.7 grams
- Hazelnuts: 2 grams
- Macadamia: 1.5 grams
- Pecans: 1.2 grams
- Pistachios: 5 grams
- Walnuts: 2 grams
- Broccoli
- Extra-virgin olive oil
- Flaxseeds
- Apple cider vinegar
- Strawberries
- Garlic

- Squash
- Shirataki noodles

Type 2 diabetes diet:

- Brown rice
- Whole wheat
- Quinoa
- Steel-cut oatmeal
- Vegetables
- Fruits
- Beans
- Lentils

Hypertension:

Avoid: Salt, Spieses, Alcohol

What to Eat:

To increase the amounts of natural potassium, magnesium, and fiber you take in, select from the following:

- apples
- apricots
- bananas
- beet greens
- broccoli
- carrots
- collards
- green beans
- dates
- grapes
- green peas
- kale
- lima beans
- mangoes
- melons

- oranges
- peaches
- pineapples
- potatoes
- raisins
- spinach
- squash
- strawberries
- sweet potatoes
- tangerines
- tomatoes
- tuna
- yogurt (fat-free)
- Leafy greens
- Garlic
- Oats
- Olive oil

Cardiovascular disease (Heart diseases):

- Avariety of fruits and vegetables,
- whole grains,
- low-fat dairy products,
- Skinless poultry and non-fried fish.
- Nuts and legumes.
- Non-tropical vegetable oils.
- Fresh or frozen vegetables and fruits
- Low-sodium canned vegetables
- Canned fruit packed in juice or water
- Coconut
- Vegetables with creamy sauces
- Fried or breaded vegetables
- Canned fruit packed in heavy syrup
- Frozen fruit with sugar added

Cancer: Constipation by drinking water and eating high-fiber foods like beans, lentils, vegetables, and **fresh** or dried fruit. Drive away diarrhea with **bland** foods such as rice, bananas, and apples.

- Carrots, peppers and greens
- Ginger
- Seeds
- Sunflower Seeds
- Pumpkin Seeds
- Sesame Seeds
- Tomatoes
- Green leafy vegetables
- Broccoli
- Garlic
- Beetroot

<u>Obesity & Weight:</u> 11 foods to avoid when you're trying to lose weight.

- French Fries and Potato Chips. Whole potatoes are healthy and filling, but french fries and potato chips are not. ...
- Sugary Drinks. ...
- White Bread. ...
- Candy Bars. ...
- Most Fruit Juices. ...
- Pastries, Cookies and Cakes. ...
- Some Types of Alcohol (Especially Beer) ...
- Ice Cream.
- Pizza & Fast foods
- High-Calorie Coffee Drinks

<u>Hypercholesterolemia:</u> Avoid these foods

- Animal products
- Butter
- Egg yolks

- High fat dairy products,chees,and whole milk yougurt
- Tropical oils, like coconut,palm oil etc.. and fried fast food
- Margarine
- Ready made baked goods, and frosted cakes
- Cake mixes
- Frozen foods. Such as pizza and pie crust
- Boxed crackers
- Donuts
- Canned and frozen biscuits
- Packaged cookies
- Candy
- Microwave popcorn

Osteoporosis:

- Dairy - milk, yoghurt, cream, cheese etc.
- Green leafy vegetables such as cabbage, broccoli, kale and okra also fennel, spinach.
- Fortified orange juice.
- Sesame seeds.
- Dried figs and apricots.

Pregnancy:

- Dairy products. During **pregnancy**, you need to consume extra protein and calcium to meet the needs of the growing fetus.
- Legumes. ...
- Sweet potatoes. ...
- Salmon. ...
- Eggs. ...
- Broccoli and dark, leafy greens. ...
- Lean meat. ...
- Fish liver oil.
- Berries
- Whole grains

- Avocados
- Dried fruit
- Water

Kidney disease:

Eat this ... (lower-potassium foods)

- Apples, cranberries, grapes, pineapples and strawberries
- Cauliflower, onions, peppers, radishes, summer squash, lettuce
- Pita, tortillas and white breads
- Beef and chicken, white rice

Rather than ... (higher-potassium foods)

- Avocados, bananas, melons, oranges, prunes and raisins
- Artichokes, winter squash, plantains, spinach, potatoes and tomatoes
- Bran products and granola
- Beans (baked, black, pinto, etc.), brown or wild rice

Eat this ... (lower-phosphorous foods)

- Italian, French or sourdough bread
- Corn or rice cereals and cream of wheat
- Unsalted popcorn
- Some light-colored sodas and lemonade

Rather than ... (higher-phosphorous foods)

- Whole-grain bread
- Bran cereals and oatmeal
- Nuts and sunflower seeds
- Dark-colored colas

Improve metabolic syndrome:

Fibrous foods include:

- fresh and frozen fruit
- dried fruit
- fresh and frozen vegetables
- oats
- barley

- dried beans
- lentils
- brown rice
- quinoa
- couscous
- bran
- whole-grain bread and pasta
- cinnamon powder

High-potassium foods to your diet:

- bananas
- dates
- orange
- grapefruit
- cantaloupe
- collard greens
- edamame beans
- black beans
- lentils
- mushrooms
- potato with skin
- tomatoes
- oat bran
- yogurt

You may benefit from the following supplements:

- **For blood sugar:** chromium supplements

- **For cholesterol:** psyllium fiber, niacin or vitamin B-3 complex supplements, omega-3 fatty acid supplements

- **For blood pressure:** potassium supplements

- **For blood pressure and cholesterol:** garlic supplements.

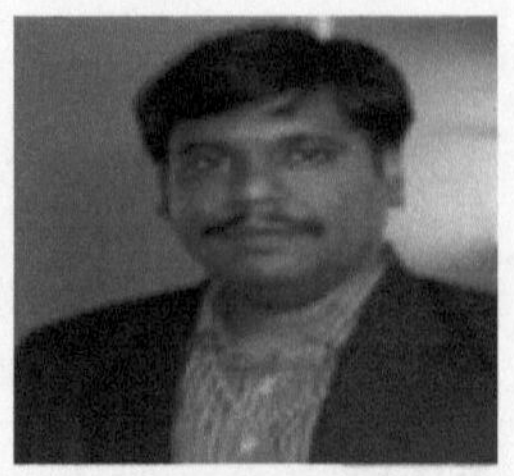

Name of the Author: Dr. Balaji Deekshitulu P V

Present working:

Homeopathy&Alt.Medi Physician& Counseling Psychologist

Educational Qualifications:
D.H.M.S, B.A.S.M, MSc (Psy), PhD, Dlitt (USA)

Published Articles:
Published **44** Research Articles.

Published Books:

- Emergency Treatment for Homeopathy

- Alternative Remedies for Stress

- Build your self

Awards

- Received PesalaNarayana Reddy Memorial Award,2012 by Bhartiya Kala Parishad, Pamoor, PrakasamDist.A.P
- Received Silver Medal in Kanchi Kama KotiPeetham
- Received Public Relations Best programmers National Award 2010, PRSI, Delhi.
- Received best Homeopathy Practitioners Award, 2011 in Homeopathic foundation, Chennai.

- Second Best elocution Prize in Sri Ramakrishna SevaSamithi, Tirupati.
- Presented by Justice M.N.Venkatachaliah, second best prize in Elocution, 1998 in the Sri Venkateswara University, Tirupati.
- Presented by KuladipNayar, M.P, Rajyasabha, first best prize in Essay writing, 1998 in the Sri Venkateswara University, Tirupati.
- Received first best prize in Elocution the SNDT women's University, Mumbai in 1999.
- Presented by Justice J.S.Verma, second best prize in Elocution, 2000 in the Sri Venkateswara University, Tirupati.
- Presented by Justice Dr.A.S.Anand Chief Justice of India, First best prize in Elocution, 2001 in the Sri Venkateswara University, Tirupati.
- 1993 Special Awarded in the elocution by Forrest department, AP state Government.
- 2008 National youth day, Govt of A.P, Second Best Prize in Elocution.
- Received by best homeo physician Obstetrics and gynaecological society, Tirupati.